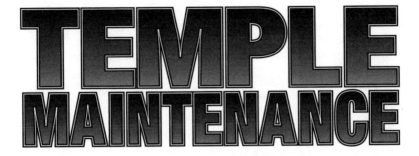

# TEMPLE MAINTENANCE

## Excellence With Love

## James P. Gills, M.D.
### & James Pitzer Gills III
#### with HeartLight

# Other Books & Materials
## by James P. Gills, M.D.
## & HeartLight

### The Unseen Essential: A Story For Our Troubled Times
ISBN 1-879938-05-7
A compelling contemporary novel about one man's journey toward God's kind of love

### Come Unto Me
ISBN 1-879938-00-6
Inspired by Dr. Gills' trip to the Holy Land, it explores God's eternal desire for mankind to get to know Him intimately

### The Dynamics of Worship
ISBN 1-879938-03-0
Designed to rekindle the heart with a passionate love for God. Gives the who, what, when, where, why and how of worship

### Love: Fulfilling the Ultimate Quest
ISBN 1-879938-02-2
A quick "refresher course" on the meaning and method of God's great gift

### The Missing Link
(No ISBN)
In a colorful, 4" x 9" pamphlet, gives the key to a joyous, faith-filled life

### Transform Your Marriage
ISBN 1-879938-11-1
An elegant 4" x 9" booklet to help couples develop new closeness with each other and with the Lord

### Tender Journey
ISBN 1-879938-17-0
The long-awaited sequel to *The Unseen Essential*

### The Prayerful Spirit
ISBN 1-879938-10-3
(by Gills with Saunders and Krueger)
Tells how prayer has changed Dr. Gills' life, the lives of patients and other doctors

### Believe and Rejoice
ISBN 1-879938-13-8
(by Gills with Krueger)
Changed by Faith, Filled with Joy

## *Dedicated to the patients I love ...and your loved ones, too.*

You are your own best physician! By simply reading this book and following the suggestions outlined within, you can practice preventive medicine. Your entire life will change if you only receive some of the wisdom accumulated from many experts in total wellness. Adapt slowly to change, but with a determination to pursue a disciplined, Christian lifestyle. Dependence on Jesus Christ is the key.

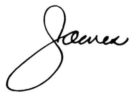 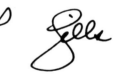

James P. Gills, M.D.

*"Do you not know that your body is a temple of the Holy Spirit, who is in you, whom you have received from God? You are not your own; you were bought with a price. Therefore honor God with your body."*

**1 Corinthians 6:19-20**

Unless otherwise indicated, Scripture references are from the **New American Standard Bible,** © The Lockman Foundation 1960, 1962, 1963, 1968, 1971, 1972, 1973, 1975, 1977. Used by permission.

Scripture references marked AMP are from **The Amplified Bible,** Old Testament © 1965, 1987 by The Zondervan Corporation. The Amplified New Testament © 1968, 1987 by The Lockman Foundation. Used by permission.

Quotation from **GETTING THIN** by Gabe Mirkin, M.D. Copyright © 1983 by Gabe Mirkin, M.D. By permission of Little, Brown and Company.

Produced by HeartLight

Typesetting by Typo-Graphics, Inc., Orlando, Florida.
Set in 12 point Cheltenham with 22 point Helvetica Bold Condensed heads.

**TEMPLE MAINTENANCE**
© 1989 by James P. Gills, M.D.
Published by LOVE PRESS:
A ministry of St. Luke's Cataract and Laser Institute
Tarpon Springs, Florida
Printed in the United States of America
First Edition: 60,000
Second Edition: 100,000
Third printing: 100,000
Fourth printing: 100,000
Fifth printing: 100,000

ISBN 1-879938-01-4

# CONTENTS

# Acknowledgements

We extend our sincere thanks to HeartLight for writing, editing, design assistance, and publishing management of LOVE PRESS since 1986. Deep appreciation goes to Bud and Pat Hamm, Distribution Managers. Also a special thank you to the many professionals who contributed anecdotes and technical information to *Temple Maintenance*. This book has been very well-received around the world. You helped to make that possible. God bless you all!

# 1 EYE-OPENING TEMPLE TOUR

# 1. You Say You Aren't Motivated?

*Dream a little... just for a moment, would you?*

*It could be you* in the historic New England city of Boston, where warm and sunny or brisk and cloudy springtime weather greets her annual Patriot's Day guests. Colorful crowds anticipating the world-reknowned 26.2-mile race make their way through the maze of centuries-old streets and begin to line the sides of the route. But wait. You're not among the 100,000 spectators. Far away at the starting line in the quaint, rural village of Hopkinton, crammed with contenders doing warm-up stretches on the Green, it's you—ready to run the oldest marathon in the United States, the famous Boston Marathon. Suddenly, you're off, in a sea of humanity on the move.

"Go, go, you can do it!" a stranger along the way cheers you on. Arms churn smoothly and leg muscles ripple their steady rhythm, alternately knotted and bunched from driving, then relaxed and flowing while reaching ahead. Each seemingly effortless stride covers the miles of ondulating countryside....

Route 135 from Hopkinton Green...past the old railroad station in Ashland...beautiful Natick...past the reservoir... branching off on Route 16...Wellesley College and its enthusiastic cheering section...the infamous turn at the fire station on Commonwealth Avenue in Newton...four hills are coming soon now...you cover the up and back down of

Heartbreak Hill without a hint of wasted motion... muscles and lungs are burning... past Boston College and the reservoir... Chestnut Hill Avenue... Cleveland Circle... Beacon Street... Kenmore Square... Commonwealth Avenue again... Hereford Street... Boylston Street... pushing hard for the remaining 600 yards... Copley Plaza Hotel, Trinity Church and the library are coming into view....

Finally, thirty yards from the finish line and still running strong. Now just ten yards to go. Already a sense of accomplishment builds, increasing with every heartbeat. And such a strong heart. Like the powerful throb of a finely-tuned engine, it sends blood coursing and keeps air flowing. Two strides left... one... the race is over! Exhilaration, joy and satisfaction, mixed with relief, push fatigue aside. What a moment!

There was a time about twenty-five years ago when I could only imagine the excitement and challenge dedicated runners felt. Now I know for myself. My own love of the sport started when, as a medical resident at Johns Hopkins University, I went running with a friend to ease the tension of school.

Today as I relax here at home, making final edits to this new edition of *Temple Maintenance,* I am reminded of my eighteenth Boston Marathon, only weeks away. Time passes so quickly. In preparation for the annual event, I've stepped up my training regimen of diet and exercise. Peaceful fatigue lingers from this afternoon's long training run of twenty-one miles. At least it's over for the week. Even though I have never come close to winning a marathon (in fact, I usually bring up the rear), just being able to finish is enough for me.

Amid a busy professional and personal schedule, I have learned to make time for good health. You can, too. Running marathons may never be your personal choice of exercise, but you can still commit yourself to taking care of your temple. That's my goal for this book. To get you "fired up for total fitness."

Mankind has always admired the superior athlete—maybe too much so. But greatness is sometimes wrapped in unexpected packages. You don't have to be twenty to pursue an exercise program. You can be over sixty, in fact. A sixty-five year-old woman came into the office of Dr. Ray Wunderlich, a brilliant doctor with a preventive medicine practice in St. Petersburg, and inspired him more than anyone during his entire medical career.

"I have a pain here on the top of my foot," she told him as she indicated the sore spot. Dr. Wunderlich noticed that the joints in her hands and feet were gnarled and bent from rheumatoid arthritis.

"How long have you had arthritis?" he asked.

"Forty years."

"Why would you come to me, a specialist in preventive medicine, with a pain in your foot?" was his next, slightly impatient question. He couldn't help thinking that aches and pains were a common complaint among people her age, especially those with arthritis.

"Well, doctor, I walk five miles every day and I don't want anything to jeopardize that...." Her voice trailed off.

He was stunned by her reply. Such resolve was humbling, even to a veteran distance runner like himself. How he tried to encourage many of his patients to get regular exercise—people much younger and less handicapped than she.

Years later, when I asked Ray how he felt about this courageous woman's answer, he paused thoughtfully. "I felt like a dot of dust in the presence of a great master. *Miniscule.*"

Well said. People like her are the real winners. The discipline and dedication she showed through her actions are as admirable as any athlete who wins the Boston Marathon, the Double Ironman or an Olympic Gold Medal. In fact, maybe more so. She did the best she could with what she had. Isn't that all any of us can ask of ourselves? Unfortunately, far too many Americans are out of condition. Soft, flabby bodies...minds awash in the waste waters of society...

spirits shut off from God. He calls us all to commitment, but slothfulness abounds instead.

Perhaps you are someone who has come to the point in your life where you're ready for a change. A new outlook. (If you're already on your way, good for you!) Would you like to have more energy, look better and be more productive? How about losing those extra pounds weighing you down? Have you gotten fed up with anxiety and compulsive behavior?

You may be saying, "*Yes,* I'm ready for the new me! Just tell me how to do it."

Well, that's a good start. If you acknowledge your need to change, you've made the first crucial step. Further, if you have a willingness and enthusiasm to improve, you could be halfway to the new you.

## Shaping Up

"Health is definitely a measurable quantity today," says cardiovascular surgeon, Dr. Charles Lasley, of Clearwater, Florida. Most of his life he has been a health evangelist (labeled a "fanatic" by his wife). At age sixty-nine, the lean, fit physician still runs at least thirty miles a week. A graduate of Harvard Medical School, cardiovascular surgeon for almost thirty years and the former director of health and fitness programs in Tampa Bay, he firmly believes Americans must change their lifestyle. Heart patients, especially, have modifications to make in order to benefit significantly from coronary bypass surgery.

Dr. Lasley divides physical health into the following four categories:

1. *Cardiovascular Fitness:* achieved by aerobic exercise of suitable intensity and duration to promote endurance.
2. *Strength:* attained by repetitions of range of motion exercises with weights.

3. *Flexibility and Coordination:* realized through stretching exercises, calisthenics and aerobics.
4. *Lowered Body Fat:* accomplished through a diet high in fiber and low in both sugar and fats.

Another cardiovascular surgeon and teacher, Dr. Peter Knight from the University of South Florida in Tampa, wasn't always committed to health. He has come a long way in temple maintenance and eagerly shares his fitness story:

"In about 1970 when I was in my late thirties, I really got convicted about my lifestyle. There was already enough information in the medical journals to convince me of the need for some changes. I realized that if I was going to continue to counsel heart patients, I would have to be a good example and clean up my own act. I weighed 175 pounds at only 5'8" tall, smoked cigarettes, had poor eating habits, didn't sleep very well and drank excessively. I seemed to always be in a rut, perpetually sluggish in both body and mind."

The changes Dr. Knight experienced did not come about because he disciplined his body through running. Neither was it because he quit smoking and drinking nor adopted healthy eating habits. Peter Knight achieved, and maintains, his high level of fitness because he made changes in all three areas of his life: body, mind and spirit.

"It wasn't easy," he confirms. "There I'd be, my overweight, out-of-shape body on Tampa's beautiful Bayshore Boulevard, running, jogging and walking — whatever I could manage. My family was tolerant, but nobody really understood my new habits. For a long time, I felt terrible when I was exercising. A number of months passed before my body reached the 'training effect.' Then I started to really enjoy myself."

You should see him now! He weighs 140 pounds and, at fifty-four years old, is in the best condition of his life. "I have more energy," he says. "I can handle stressful situations more positively and I rest easier. Best of all, I have an increased level of enthusiasm in all areas of my life.

"The Lord has made it easier for me to continue a wellness lifestyle," says Dr. Knight. "I've got to keep the engine tuned up to give the Lord His best day. The more mature in the Lord a person becomes and the more important his Christian walk, the greater motivating factor that is. My priorities have changed a lot. I used to be quite competitive. Now I try to be a witness.

"My biggest disappointment was that I couldn't convince my father-in-law to follow suit, no matter how hard I tried. He was a great man, an enjoyable person who had a lot to offer, but he was way overweight. He died prematurely, and there was just nothing I could do.

"On the other hand, Mayor Bill Poe of Tampa had a heart attack and stroke in the prime of his life; he couldn't even talk for awhile. When I was called in as a consulting physician, he said, 'That's it. What do I have to do?' He made up his mind and persevered. The next year he was running in the Gasparilla three-mile race."

Dr. Ken Cooper, credited by many to be the "father of the fitness boom," emphasizes the importance of those healthy changes Dr. Knight and his patient experienced in their lives. Ken summarized his position in a talk entitled, "Six Things That Affect Glorifying God's Body." They are: 1) *weight and diet* 2) *exercise* 3) *eliminating tobacco products* 4) *no alcohol or drugs* 5) *managing stress* 6) *periodic physical exams.* We'll look at each area briefly and then expand on diet and exercise in the next section.

## Weight and Diet

Dr. Cooper points out that weight and diet concerns should be reasonable. "Do you recommend fasting to lose weight?" would-be dieters often ask. According to Dr. Cooper, fasting is not a good way to lose weight. Pounds are shed by a loss in muscle tissue and upon completion of the fast, weight returns in the form of fat. The result: a continuous cycle of less muscle and more fat, making it all the more difficult to stay in shape and keep the proper weight. (Fasting periodically for spiritual reasons is another matter.)

You can determine your ideal weight by performing a relatively simple calculation. Men: multiply your height in inches by 4; then subtract 128. Women: multiply your height in inches by 3.5 and subtract 108.

For example, let's say you're a female who's 5'6" tall. With the above formula, you would multiply 66 (inches tall) x 3.5 to get 231. Then subtract 108 from 231 to arrive at your approximate ideal weight of 123 pounds. If, when you step on the bathroom scale for your weekly check-up, it registers 145, you are about twenty-two pounds, or nineteen per cent, overweight. A person could be considered obese who weighs twenty per cent or more over his or her ideal body weight. Should this be the case, it may be time to give some serious thought to a change in lifestyle.

The successful *Free to Be Thin* weight loss program, founded by 113-pound loser Neva Coyle, takes an unusual approach to finding and maintaining perfect weight. She believes prayer and the Word are the best formula. Since the Bible gives assurance that God knows your frame (He made it), He knows how much weight your body should carry to function best. When you think about it, the Lord was very specific about the dimensions of both the tabernacle in the wilderness and the temple of Solomon. Your body is a temple, too. He probably has your perfect size in mind.

Have you ever heard of "black calories?" Dr. John Verner, a wellness physician from the Watson Clinic in Lakeland, Florida, finds that many people who struggle continuously with weight control consume high amounts of those "nocturnal no-no's." "Black calories" are simply calories eaten after dark, with no chance to burn them off through work or exercise.

By the way, many people hang on for dear life to a common fallacy about fat. They think they can decrease body fat in a particular area by simply exercising that one part of the body. A good example is the woman who hopes to gain a firm, flat stomach by doing sit-ups. Unfortunately, her stomach stays fat because of an accumulation of fat cells there. The area cannot be reduced until these are eliminated through proper dieting— mainly by ridding the body of cholesterol-causing sugars and fats. Even bodybuilders can build massive muscles and still lack definition until they lower their percentage of body fat.

"The closer your diet comes to being vegetarian, the healthier and leaner you will be, and the less risk you will run of developing not only vascular disease and obesity, but also cancer," advises Dr. Verner. He presents an excellent array of ideas on health at symposiums on Executive Wellness.

## *Tobacco, Alcohol and Drugs— Deadly Enemies*

United States Surgeon General C. Everett Koop, in the 1989 study, *"Reducing the Health Consequences of Smoking: 25 Years of Progress,"* reports, "Smoking is responsible for more than one of every six deaths in the United States. Smoking remains the single most important preventable cause of death in our society."

One pack of cigarettes a day increases the chance of lung cancer to a level twenty times greater than that of non-smokers. It leads inactivity and obesity as factors that accelerate the aging process and shortens life expectancy by at least *five and a half minutes per cigarette.* Even more alarming are the problems of cardiovascular diseases, cancer of the esophagus, cancer of the pancreas and other difficult-to-treat cancers. How tragic to see coronary artery disease rising even in young women who smoke.

Advertising has spent billions of dollars trying to glamorize the "sip and puff" lifestyle in America, but don't believe a word. It is far from glamorous. Consider the experience of a man I admire tremendously, Dr. Bill Hale, from Dunedin, Florida, who suffered a heart attack at an early age. When reviewing his past habits he came to the startling conclusion that the only thing he did wrong was smoke.

Alcohol consumption has escalated to the third leading cause of death in the United States. Chronic use damages the liver, heart and brain. The National Research Council makes this recommendation about alcohol: drink none, or at most one ounce of pure alcohol per day. I say, "Stick with none." Alcohol can take twelve years off your time here on earth.

The use of alcohol and other drugs is a subtle form of self-poisoning. These substances cause many body systems to function below their optimum, due to toxicity. For example, they deplete the serotonin level in the brain, which leads to depression and inefficient mental faculties. Another side effect of substance abuse? The acceleration of the natural decline of brain tissue which begins at about eighteen years of age. These could be major contributing factors to many of the brain syndromes we find so terrifying.

Over the past thirty years, alcohol and other drug use among adolescents has become a social problem of epidemic proportions. Violence (traffic fatalities, homicide, suicide), now the major cause of death among our youth, directly relates to drug use, according to OSAP (Office for Substance Abuse Prevention). AIDS, other crime and school drop-out are closely associated, as well. On the most recent National Household Survey (1985) sponsored by the National Institute on Drug Abuse (NIDA), young drug users, especially, reported multiple symptoms from their habit such as anxiety, irritability, lower productivity and inability to think clearly.

Life may not always be a bed of roses, but why forfeit, so casually, one-sixth or more of your life? Flee these harmful substances like the plague they are. Avoid coffee and other caffeinated drinks, too. As many groups in recent years have discovered, caffeine produces irregularities in heart function, increases cholesterol levels and aggravates nervous tension.

## Stress and Exercise

Stress threatens health profoundly. Although a major aspect of life, we all handle it less optimally than we could. Effects of stress— headaches, fatigue, loss of appetite, ulcers and high blood pressure— are a drain on the entire body. While some stress proves desirable, prolonged stress often precedes the onset of many different disease complexes.

I have found my relationship with Jesus Christ to be the most effective way to relieve stress and anxiety. Faith in Him gets rid of fear. We'll explore more about spiritual maintenance in Part Four.

Regular exercise also alleviates stress. Such a program lowers the pulse response to stress to approximately one-third of what it would have been without exercise. In addition, it provides an outlet for stress-produced adrenalin, allowing you to remain calm. Secretions known as endorphins and serotonin are released in the brain during aerobic exercise and can actually help control pain and overcome depression.

Martha MacGregor, a close friend of my wife, Heather, is a vibrant lady who discovered that secret for herself. Through exercise, she found relief from "the blues." She shared with Heather, "After my father's death, I was very anxious and depressed for quite awhile. I just couldn't seem to shake it. A friend kept urging me to go jogging with her. She said I would feel so much better, but I stubbornly resisted. Finally, she almost *dragged* me along, and am I glad she did! The depression began to lift within days and I've continued jogging regularly ever since. That was nine years ago."

Beneficial exercise should be geared to individual needs and abilities without being excessive (I can't say I've been too diligent on that one.) Speaking of overdoing it, that reminds me of Jackson Hole, Wyoming in 1985. I was in the mood for some serious skiing. Would you believe... that tram carried me up on every single 4139 vertical-foot trip it made from early morning until early afternoon? I'd race down the slopes to beat the twelve-minute tram and then ride back to the top—a total of about 65,000 vertical feet. It was fun for the time. When I had to nurse second degree burns on my face and a body full of screaming muscles, the fun wore off in a hurry, however. Two weeks later, I had just about recovered. So, moderation does have its value, if sometimes dull.

Running flashes another yellow caution light. If you are running more than fifteen miles per week, consider your goals carefully. Dr. Cooper recommends that the average person run no more than fifteen miles per week to avoid leg problems and other injuries. Some experts feel that burning 2000 calories a week through exercise is ideal. That's the equivalent of running twenty miles, biking one hundred miles or swimming four to five miles.

I have found, after adapting to long distance running for over twenty years, that seventy miles a week is the best amount for me. Besides making me a stronger competitor, it helps me feel better, control my weight, relieve tension, be more tranquil and mentally alert. Any exercise routine will provide greater health rewards if rounded out with other sports.

## Physical Exams

Finally, Ken Cooper emphasizes the importance of periodic physical exams. A routine physical, with blood studies and stress tests, should be done at regular intervals throughout your life. In this way, certain cancers and other troublesome syndromes may be detected early enough to be treated and eradicated completely. Your physician may also discover the early warning signs of heart trouble. Many people are not aware of advanced cardiovascular disease because there are no symptoms; a heart attack may be the first sudden, and often fatal sign.

Are you planning to begin an exercise program, even a mild one? I sure hope so ... you won't regret it. Have a thorough physical examination by a qualified doctor first. Dr.

Verner from the Watson Clinic gives some guidelines about what to expect from a good physical exam. Each one should be composed of three specific areas: *evaluation, education* and *motivation.*

The evaluation stage provides the physician with information on your current lifestyle, family background (for potentially weak genes), medical history and personal goals. This will include the physical exam and numerous tests. In the area of education, the physician compiles all the information gleaned from the evaluation to determine where you need to modify your habits—what you should delete and what you should add.

Motivation may come from the physician who actually follows his own prescriptions. Not only can he advise you what to do, he can testify to the rewards you will reap from your efforts. And the old adage still rings true: "An ounce of prevention is worth a pound of cure."

# 2. Excellence, With Love

**W**hat state is your temple in? Does it require major renovation, or are you the kind of meticulous caretaker who maintains a sure foundation? Is it strong, free of creaking, misshapen bones, and supported by lean, pliable muscles? How about the "air-conditioning" and "plumbing?" Will they get you to the finish line?

An uninhabitable temple is of little use. Superficial facades cannot hide poor inner maintenance for very long. On the other hand, if the rooms have been properly cared for, this, too, will be evident. Air will circulate freely, pumped by the main compressor—a strong, vigorous heart—through a network of unclogged blood vessels. Physical activity can only change your outward appearance by toning the muscles within. Modified eating habits will enhance your physique by eliminating underlying fat.

This principle (the outside reflects what's inside) applies consistently throughout each major area of life. In much the same way that well-cared-for organs radiate health to those who meet you, a strong relationship with God creates an air of serenity by establishing peace and joy within. *"By wisdom a house is built, and by understanding it is established; and by knowledge the rooms are filled with all precious and pleasant riches,"* says Proverbs 24:3,4. You build a temple fit for the Master's use the same way.

"I never dreamed I could look and feel like this at my age! Not only that—things are starting to go better at work and with the family. Now that my priorities are straightened out, I'm much more satisfied in life. After all these years, it's great to know where I'm going."

Such a testimony could easily have been my own when I began a serious temple maintenance regimen in my late twenties. I'm still able to say it in my fifties, thank the Lord. You can make it your own personal testimony, too. I firmly believe that anyone who will pursue the suggestions outlined in this book can achieve significant, fulfilling results.

There is a certain *"rightness"* about being healthy. True health goes far beyond the physical to encompass clear mental faculties and a spirit in love with its Creator. While the body, mind and spirit can theoretically be separated, they are one. They work together as a team. Actually, you *are* a spirit; you *have* a soul; you *live* in a body. Only when all three areas are healthy, can you be your best in any one aspect. Thus, to glorify God and enjoy life to the fullest, a good temple maintenance program encompasses all three—body, mind and spirit.

Of what use is it to be in peak physical condition, if your mind is so uncontrolled that you find concentrating on one task impossible for more than a few minutes at a time? Or if your spirit is so out of tune with God that you are void of a reason to live? Commitment to disciplined excellence is your calling in life. *Excellence, with love*.

One business associate who desired to make such a commitment asked me how I became a disciplined person. (Remember now, any strength has the potential to be a flaw. Just ask my wife, Heather.)

"Did a crisis occur in your life to force you to become so dedicated to temple maintenance or have you always been that way?" she wanted to know.

"Habit," I answered. "It started with the way I grew up. My father and grandfather were very self-disciplined. At thirteen years of age I had my own business taking out garbage, cutting grass and delivering newspapers. My father could afford to give me money, but he felt it wasn't the best thing for me. I was always involved in sports, too."

"Why do you feel people are so undisciplined today?" was her next question.

"Society has changed," I philosophized. "A story I heard provides a good example. The professor stormed into his classroom in a fit of frustration and wrote **'APATHY!'** in huge letters on the blackboard. One student leaned over to his classmate and whispered, 'What does apathy mean?'

*'Who cares?'* came the reply.

"That's the problem. So few care. Work isn't as important anymore, either. Many employees take no pride in what they do. They want to get without giving. Back when I was growing up, a man's self-worth was based on his responsible and dependable behavior.

"I especially remember a Sunday School teacher who had a profound effect on me when I was a young boy. I admired him greatly and wanted to be like him. Not only was he an athlete—a college boxer—he was an intelligent businessman and a fantastic teacher. He taught with so much life and put everything he had into everything he did. But, people had more respect back then for authority figures and teachers. A lack of respect goes with a lack of discipline," I concluded.

She pressed me further in her quest for temple maintenance. "If slothfulness is sin, as the Bible says, what about all those of us who didn't grow up with the self-discipline you did? For us it *isn't* habit. Are we doomed forever to a disorganized, unhealthy lifestyle? What hope do we have of overcoming the sin of laziness and developing habits that will lead to total fitness?" She needed answers.

Well, I would say to her, and to you, that I believe in hope for lasting change, for one reason. The Gospel is a message of hope. *"I can do all things through Christ, who strengthens me."* Dependence on Him has been my secret. His Spirit will guide you, too, and produce good fruit in every area of your life. More about the "how-to" of that concept will be coming in Part Four.

## The Responsibility Factor

It's never too late to achieve rewards from healthy habits, no matter how old you are when you start. Results are noticed more quickly at a younger age, but you still owe it to yourself and your family to be your strongest and healthiest—not just for this life, but for the life eternal.

If you are stuck in the rut of smoking, drinking, poor diet, inactivity, unwholesome thought patterns or separation from God, think through the final results of your lifestyle. Yes, you may feel that it's your life and you can do what you want with it, but what about your spouse? Your children? As bad habits take their toll, family members are the ones who must ultimately compensate for your inability to care for yourself physically and financially, a burden that may continue for many years. The consequences of a reckless lifestyle don't always lead to sudden death.

Dr. Charles Lasley encourages,

We have arrived at a point in our collective awareness about health and risk factors that each of us must assume some individual responsibility for our lifestyle and develop positive additions or health habits to lessen these risk factors. We may say that we don't want to pay the price it takes to achieve this kind of cardiovascular fitness and super health. That is, avoiding the toxic drugs— tobacco, alcohol, caffeine, staying away from fats and sugars, eating raw fiber foods and getting a minimum of thirty to forty minutes of vigorous aerobic exercise most days. That is our informed choice to make, but it is most important that we know the difference between one lifestyle and the other. We must not only realize the difference of methods of achievement, but more importantly, the difference in results.

Dr. Peter Knight also emphasizes personal accountability in an article for a local medical journal. He quotes the late John Knowles,

> Prevention of disease means forsaking the bad habits which many people enjoy—overeating, too much drinking, staying up at night, engaging in promiscuous sex, driving too fast, and smoking cigarettes . . . The cost of sloth, gluttony, alcoholic intemperance, reckless driving, sexual frenzy, and smoking is now a national, and not an individual responsibility. This is justified as individual freedom— but one man's freedom in health is another man's shackle in taxes and in insurance premiums. I believe the idea of a "right" to health should be replaced by the idea of an individual moral obligation to preserve one's own health—a public duty, if you will.

The most poignant example of the question of responsibility vs. personal freedom was in a story I heard some time ago. A gentleman was sharing his agony over a tragedy in his family. For years, he strongly urged his wife when they rode in the car, "Will you please wear your seat belt?" She told him, "No, it's *my* life and *I'll* decide whether or not to wear one." Now she is paralyzed from a serious car accident. Since then, it is all he can do to keep from despising her for her short-sightedness; only Jesus can help him forgive. He has a major responsibility in caring for his invalid wife. Plans they had for their life together have been drastically changed because of her selfishness.

Was it *really* this woman's life to ruin as she pleased? Did she have a right to ruin his, as well? A Christian has an additional responsibility because his body was bought with a costly price—the blood of Jesus Christ. Your temple is not your own. It is His.

## Sticking With It

I believe if you could catch hold of one basic truth, it wouldn't be such a battle to conjure up the motivation and discipline to care for your temple. You see, as sobering as all the results of neglect are, they only wake you up to reality for a moment. You soon forget. Or even as wonderful as all the benefits of optimum health are—feeling good, looking better, losing weight, gaining energy and handling stress well—they are not enough reasons for you to be persistent, either. For the most part, they are only self-gratifying. Humanistic, self-centered motivation falls short in the long run. You can work under a higher law, and respond to a loftier calling. *Love.*

Love is the first and highest commandment, Jesus said. Love fulfills the law, wrote the Apostle Paul. In other words, love in your heart can get you to do what no amount of external rules and prodding and brow-beating can. You can read hundreds of books on fitness (there are probably that many), go to diet classes, exercise regularly, read the Bible and countless religious books. You may even see some results, but none of it will bring you lasting joy. Freedom will still elude you.

But . . . what if your decision to finally take care of your temple, God's home, springs forth out of exhuberant love for Him and His people (you, included)? If love for Jesus Christ, residing in the deepest recesses of your heart, motivates you, you won't want to quit. When you realize His commitment of love to you remains steadfast for eternity, that love will forge a lifetime commitment in you. Dependent love for Jesus Christ will instill godly discipline in you, even if you possess little to none right now. Trust Him to bring it to pass. He is more than able.

Thousands of years ago lived a Hebrew man named Joseph who was motivated by love during a very difficult test of self-discipline. You may remember that his jealous brothers had thrown him in a pit and watched as he was sold into slavery. His new Egyptian boss, Potiphar, perceived Joseph's outstanding character and eventually entrusted him to manage everything he owned. Then the drama really began. Potiphar's beautiful, lustful wife invited the handsome, well-built Joseph to go to bed with her. His answer spoke volumes about him, *"How can I do such a wicked thing as this? It would be a great sin against God"* (Genesis 39:8,9).

Wouldn't that have been a desirable offer for a young, virile, unmarried man? But love and respect for his earthly master as well as his heavenly One kept Joseph pure. His restraint resulted from more than just having memorized the seventh commandment, *"Thou shalt not commit adultery"* (Exodus 20:14). Love, the first commandment, held him back.

He didn't treat Potiphar's brazen wife with disrespect when she kept after him. He even had to tell her "no" several times. Yes, he did pay dearly for his godly choice. He was sent to prison after she, in probable retaliation from the bruise to her feminine ego, falsely accused him of rape.

Joseph survived. Discipline born of love stood him in good stead throughout his years as a slave and prisoner, eventually allowing him to be promoted to second in command over all of Egypt. Discipline born of love helped him to be open to divine wisdom for a plan. God used him to save the world of his day from starvation by famine.

Like Joseph, hasn't your Creator and Master given *you* charge over all He owns, especially your temple? When the temptations of lust, gluttony, and slothfulness come to seduce you, as they no doubt will, love for your Master, yourself and those around you, will cause you to triumph. He who is the same yesterday, today, and forever, promises a way of escape from every temptation. Victory in Jesus!

The words to a poem written by my editors, HeartLight, sum up the motivation to which I encourage you: *excellence, with love*.

"My body is a temple,
The Spirit dwells within.
He wants me to maintain it
And guard it from sin,

To keep it pure and holy,
Clean and undefiled.
*I'll do it because I love Him,*
*'Cause I am God's child.*
Temple maintenance, temple maintenance!"

Throughout the rest of **Temple Maintenance,** we will delve more deeply into each area of fitness mentioned so far: physical, mental and spiritual. Part Two, maintenance of the body, concentrates on exercise and diet, with many variations on a theme. In Part Three, we will examine what is sometimes referred to as the soul—the mental aspect of your temple. We'll look at the mind's potential and then break it down into bite-sized pieces of intellect, emotions and will, along with a host of ideas about how to maintain them in peak condition.

Part Four encompasses a discussion of your spirit. You'll learn a great deal about your spirit and its unique functions— communion, conscience and intuition—as well as how to keep in shape there, too.

"I agree that body, mind and spirit work together," you might be thinking. "But if the spirit is most important, why not discuss it first?" That's a good question. Maybe it's wise to save the best for last, the most critical ideas for the most-remembered time. Then again, sometimes it's just easier to start with what you can see and touch and move on to the invisible realm. Jesus did in His earthly ministry. Still, there could be a more profound reason.

When God created man, He first made his physical body out of the dust of the earth and then breathed life into him. Also, do you recall the tabernacle in the wilderness and later, Solomon's temple? They were designed so that first came the outer court, then the holy place and finally, the holy of holies.

Each of those three areas of the ancient temple seems to correspond to the human temple: outer court/physical body, holy place/mind, and holy of holies/spirit. The parts of the tabernacle all lend deeper insight into how your temple should function. In the Old Testament, the high priest passed through one area in order to reach the other. He began first in the outer court, moved on to the holy place and finally once a year, entered the holy of holies. So it "feels" right to begin now with the body, progress to the mind and end with the spirit. We'll look further at the correlation between old and new temples in Part Five.

Also in Part Five you'll see how body, mind and spirit should work as a balanced team. You will evaluate your current temple wellness, and set your sights for the future so you can get your own program off the ground. We have filled the book with personal experiences of my own and others, for your reading pleasure. Such is your road map to *Temple Maintenance.* Enjoy the rest of the trip!

# 2

## LIFE IN THE OUTER COURT: YOUR BODY

# 3. Exercise, the Endless Energizer

"Caught up in the fitness craze, I joined a club that offered a reasonably priced membership. Although I never went, a year later I hurried back to renew. 'Do you guys have a name for people like me who join and never show up?' I jokingly asked the well-muscled man behind the counter.

'Sure,' he responded with a grin. *'Profit.'*"[1]
—Randy Padawer in ***Reader's Digest***

As funny as this little story may be, you desire a higher goal for your exercise program than merely lining the pockets of the fitness industry. Your goal is better health. Right? But you fight natural laws when you decide to get in shape. In the science of physics, the law of inertia states that a body at rest tends to stay at rest. Have you noticed? The toughest part of exercise is simply getting started. That's why so many people never do.

According to marathon runner and author George Sheehan, exercise deficiency is undoubtedly the most prevalent cause of ill health in America. Whether you are twenty-five, thirty-five, or even ninety-five years old, you can be physically fit. If not, you are settling for less than you deserve. Even more tragic: exercise deficiency is a self-inflicted disease. What an old, familiar story— man's tendency to cheat on himself. Wrongfully, he thinks he can enjoy all the fullness of life without paying a price, but he finally learns that neither the world nor the human machine works that way.

My wife, Heather, shares these thoughts from her experience with regular exercise,

> The older you get the more you have to make yourself do it, and the longer you go without it, the harder it is to get back. Many people set aside two or three days a week to exercise, but something always comes up at least one out of three days. That leaves only two, or maybe one day, which just isn't enough. A more realistic goal is to plan on exercising every day for at least thirty minutes. Then you're held accountable to yourself and the program.

> Accountability is so important to exercise. We learned the truth of this when St. Luke's sponsored free, professionally-instructed aerobics classes for our staff. Classes were offered on the second floor of St. Luke's at 4:00 p.m. and 5:00 p.m., three times a week. Initially, about fifty women expressed an interest in aerobics. After four months, only a handful were still going. Then we decided to pay only half of the instructor's fee and let the class members share the other half. They began encouraging one another to go, because the fee would be lower when divided among more people. Now, the exercise class has higher numbers again and they are reaping the benefits of fitness.

> Two or three assistants who work in the operating room with Dr. Gills are the exception; they require little outside prodding. When all surgical patients have gone—sometimes late in the evening—these ladies borrow St. Luke's video machine and work out together to a tape. Most of us are not that motivated, so it helps us to do things like 1) Promise someone to go; 2) Pay a yearly membership fee; 3) Pay for a class; 4) Invest in some

equipment. You've got to have a reason to exercise, even if it's just for enjoyment.

I personally like a lot of options and variety in my regimen, a concept explained well by Ken and Millie Cooper in their book, *The New Aerobics for Women.* They incorporate a balance of flexibility and commitment. I try to do some type of exercise every day. For me, it's a combination of playing tennis once a week for fun, biking twelve miles to St. Luke's three mornings while Jimmy runs (not much of an aerobic exercise, but great for the derriere), walking a fast three miles the other days and working out on weight machines in between. I purposely choose situations I get "locked into," like taking Jimmy's eighty-nine year-old mother to Total Fitness Center in Tarpon Springs. I know she's waiting for me, and that helps me to maintain my commitment.

Fitness miracles do happen when individuals commit themselves to wise exercise programs. The human body adapts extremely well to conditioning; a physically fit body is capable of endurance and speed far beyond present conceptions. In all sports, athletes break records continually as new physical training techniques are developed. Underlying all exercise regimens should be the following ten purposes. Do any of these benefits appeal to you? They're yours, for the working:

1. Promote general health and well-being for work and family
2. Lower the percentage of body fat
3. Help achieve proper weight
4. Insure cardiovascular conditioning
5. Gain muscle flexibility
6. Increase muscle tone and strength
7. Improve coordination
8. Provide enjoyment

9. Complement other exercises and sports
10. Enhance God's temple for more meaningful purposes

## The Get Ready, Get Set, Go! Warm-up

Adequate warm-up stimulates blood flow to the muscles and is essential to prepare the body for any athletic endeavor, especially strenuous activity. How about a warm shower? That's a good way to start the process, and next should come some stretching exercises. Stiff muscles find relief and blood flow increases further. Stretch before and after all forms of exercise.

For several months, I decreased stretching time and paid dearly for it with a disabling, tight hamstring. Following this setback, I started stretching strenuously and got back into my previous form. It seems that a good warm-up time is especially important for those of us who run high mileage, or who are advancing in years. Some athletes I know regard stretching as a waste of time, so they never do it. We're all unique, aren't we?

If you're a newcomer to exercise, you'd do better to be safe than sorry. Most experts stress the need for beginning at a moderate pace before moving into all-out exertion. Warming up is not a time-waster...you'll be glad you did, and your body will thank you for it. So, S-T-R-E-T-C-H!

Here are a couple of other pre-exercise tips. Try to avoid eating a lot of solid foods before a long or strenuous work-out. You'll need to build up fluid, sugar, and electrolytes (positive/negative ions in solution; a balance of sodium and potassium) in drinks like "Gatorade." Aspirin and other non-steroidal anti-inflammatory agents such as Motrin and Nuprin may be helpful before prolonged, intense sessions to minimize pain, muscle spasms or even plain old sore muscles.

## Aerobic Exercise for A Happy, Healthy Heart

"Aerobics is a series of strenuous exercises which help convert fats, sugars and starches into aches, pains and cramps," quipped *Mature Living* magazine. Although a small price-tag accompanies aerobic exercise, it provides so many advantages, I don't have enough space to elaborate upon them in the confines of these few pages. Your cardiovascular system will reap the most noticeable benefits from aerobics, but your entire temple will improve also. This type of exercise can decrease angina by stimulating blood flow around blocked vessels in the heart, as well as by improving the function and efficiency of existing healthy fibers in the cardiac muscle.

Aerobic exercise actually lowers blood pressure by strengthening the heart in this way, reports Dr. Knight and other cardiologists. Consequently, the incidence of stroke, heart and kidney failure lessens. "In a mild case of hypertension, regular aerobics gives a fifty/fifty chance of eliminating high blood pressure medication, or at least decreasing it," says Dr. Knight. That's good news!

"Heart-building" exercises comprise those fun aerobic sports that lead to the highest degree of fitness. Ultimately, they increase the efficient use of oxygen by the heart and lungs. The goal of aerobics, as Dr. Verner from the Watson Clinic so eloquently states it, "is to push yourself for a sustained period at a rate just short of a stitch in the side three times a week." Think F.I.T.— *frequency, intensity and time.*

The pulse is a good measuring stick. It should rise to a rate of between 130 and 150 beats per minute (or more depending upon fitness) and remain there for about twenty to thirty minutes. To determine just where to aim, use the following simple steps adapted from Dr. Cooper's book, ***The Aerobics Program for Total Well-Being.***

1. Take your resting heart rate per minute. Check your pulse, preferably at the heart itself or at the wrist, for fifteen seconds and multiply that number by four. (He feels fifteen seconds gives a more accurate reading than six or ten seconds.)
2. Find your predicted maximum heart rate (PMHR). Men: 205 minus 1/2 your age. Women: 220 minus 1/2 your age.

3. Multiply that number (PMHR) by .80 to determine where your heart rate should be during exercise. In other words, you should work out at about eighty per cent of the maximum heart rate for your age, or at least in the range of seventy-five to eighty-five per cent of your maximum.

Let's try an example to make it easier. For the moment, say you're a forty-two year-old man ready to start a running program. First, you want to know the number of heartbeats per minute you should maintain for a good workout, but yet, a number below the danger zone. One-half your age is twenty-one, so subtract that from 205. Did you get 184? Then multiply 184 by .80 to arrive at 147. In order to receive an aerobic training effect, you'll have to achieve a heart rate of 147 beats per minute for at least twenty minutes, four times a week.

I often wear a pulse monitor that attaches to my wrist and chest, and I'd recommend it for any serious trainers. A good one costs about two hundred dollars, but eliminates the potential for error when you try to monitor your heart rate during exercise. That's because you have to stop somewhat to count and your heart rate starts to slow down immediately. Also, if you have had any cardiovascular problems, a pulse monitor assures you that your heart isn't working *too* hard.

Aerobic exercise is not limited to running, jogging or exercise albums. Swimming, walking, biking, aerobic dance classes and cross-country skiing all make excellent choices. As Dr. Verner already pointed out, you only need to exercise three times a week to maintain a high level of fitness (but more is better, of course). Unlike calories, fitness cannot be stored so you must make it a habit.

## Scheduling F.I.T. Sessions

"Choose your own best time of day to exercise," says Dr. Lasley. He admits that he has worked so hard over the years convincing people to do some type of exercise, he'll settle for any time of day. Are you a morning person? Early morning aerobics produce a feeling of well-being. They may also help you perform better at work.

Lunch-time aerobics have a few other advantages: they take no additional time from sleep and family activities. Aside from breaking up the day, lunch-time aerobics keep you from eating a heavy lunch—a sure road to a lethargic afternoon.

End-of-the-day aerobics aid in relieving stress that develops throughout the day. You may find that you sleep better, too. Take all of these factors into consideration as you decide upon your own ideal exercise schedule. If it agrees with you, you'll be more apt to be consistent.

As a precaution, no matter what time slot you choose for your workout program, begin with a realistic goal in sight. You can do more harm than good by striving immediately for your training heart rate. Cardiovascular fitness can best be achieved by starting out s-l-o-w-l-y. That means, for example, walking progressively longer distances until you build up to running, or whatever your preferred strenuous aerobic activity may be.

## The Cross-Training Advantage

"Variety is the spice of life," goes the old saying which applies nicely to a fitness program. Before settling on one specific exercise, consider cross-training, a combination of many forms of exercise such as swimming, biking, Nautilus conditioning, stretching, and jumping rope. This can enhance what could otherwise become a dull routine. As my wife mentioned, she stays better motivated this way.

In addition, supporters of cross-training list the following reasons to participate in several sports: greater flexibility, increased strength, less fatigue, improved physique, increased endurance, less susceptibility to injury, enlarged scope of competition and friends, and faster recovery from exhaustion or athletic injury. Remember to warm up thoroughly, no matter which sports you choose.

Are you interested in keeping abreast of the latest health and fitness news? You might want to join *The American Running and Fitness Association.* For a twenty-five dollar tax-deductible membership fee, they will send you their monthly newsletter covering a wide range of topics, from nutrition and weight control to cycling and weight training. For more information, write: AR & FA, 2001 S. Street, N.W., Suite 540, Washington, D.C. 20009.

## Biking is Beautiful

Cycling ranks as one of Dr. Ken Cooper's "top five" aerobic exercises. It's a great sport for developing cardiovascular endurance and building leg muscles. The joints undergo less stress than in jogging, but equipment costs more. Nevertheless, anyone's budget can work in the sport of bicycling.

A bike should be selected according to three criteria: available funds, needs, and goals. Too often, would-be bicyclists go far beyond their needs and abilities in selecting equipment. If I might say so, I think one of the reasons bikers like the sport is they enjoy owning an adult "hobby horse." Pride of ownership, or a "keeping up with the Joneses" attitude prevails. A good production bike will suffice for most people. By comparison, would it make sense to drive a Ferrari just to the convenience store and back, or a Chevette around the race track? Truthfully, the *rider* is more important than the bike.

Training techniques vary. For beginners, Dr. Cooper suggests allowing ten weeks to work up to a cruising speed of fifteen miles per hour. This figures out to be a four-minute mile. Anything faster than that, he says, is not necessary to achieve an adequate aerobic training effect. Bike training should mix both short and long rides, with speed intervals spread throughout the workout. If your goals include ultra distance of a hundred miles or more, train heavily on ultra distance, and vice versa.

With a long workout ahead, drink plenty of fluids and shift your body often to prevent soreness. You will usually share the road with motor vehicles, so make a concerted effort to obey traffic regulations: bike with the flow of traffic, use hand signals, have a rear-view mirror and be ready to go onto the shoulder of the road. By all means invest in a good crash helmet and some reflective clothing, and wear them every time you go bike riding.

One other word of advice, in case you fall. If there's a chance you might be injured, stop. After I took a tumble during a bike race in Brooksville, I kept riding and decided to finish the remaining sixty miles. It turned out I had cracked my hipbone. Those surrounding muscles took as long to relax as my hip did to heal, and I was out of commission for awhile. So, quit while you're ahead, and...happy wheeling!

## Flipped Over Swimming

Swimming is another favorite of mine. You will enjoy its two-fold advantage over other sports: it has the lowest injury rate and tones more of the different muscles throughout the body. While some people swim daily, others swim only every other day and alternate with running or biking. Most people start swimming short distances, from twenty-five yards to a quarter of a mile, and then work up to several miles in their daily routine. To familiarize yourself with the basics, check out an excellent source, James Counsilman's book, *The Science of Swimming.*

Counsilman's tips will help the novice as well as the more experienced swimmer. He suggests using a high elbow when performing the stroking motion. Such a style, with the hand held close to the body, is optimal because it allows the entire forearm to exert pressure through the water. This effective motion involves a different stroking action than the stiff arm.

Another helpful hint concerns the importance of finger position when entering the water. Holding the small finger higher than both the thumb and index finger creates a cleaner planing action. As far as the kicking motion, Counsilman says that it should be done with the feet beneath the surface of the water. Even the slightest hint of churning water over the feet signals wasted energy. You will understand the importance as you begin training.

Once you make the decision to start swimming, seek a good instructor to help you get started right. Remember, it is always easier to form good habits than to break bad ones. Try the local YMCA, an ideal place to look for a swimming instructor. They may have, or can refer you to, a Master's Program for people above the junior age group. Many YMCA's have age groups extending well into advanced years, with classes tailored to meet individual need.

Swimming in the local pool does have its advantages over navigating other, more natural bodies of water. One of my scariest moments in sports occurred almost thirty-five years ago when I was a lifeguard at Myrtle Beach. My habit was to swim a mile in the ocean each evening to keep in shape. I was not the only water-lover out there keeping in shape, however.

Who should be the uninvited guests in my path, but a school of jellyfish! I swam right through them before I even knew what happened. Ouch! It felt like they stung every inch of me. Even today when I'm training in the Gulf, I fear jellyfish more than sharks who circle around me and swim off. Various species of fish pass by and seem to check me out in my orange cap . . . fisherman have started to recognize me and wave. Such is the life of a confirmed ocean swimmer. It's adventure on the high seas.

## Running and Jogging for Joy

The recent running craze has overtaken the country. When the bug bit me way back in 1963, I was a resident at Johns Hopkins University. I was working so much that I ate everything in sight, until my weight had reached about 215 pounds. Finding relief from nervous tension was probably my main motivation to run. Late at night when I got off work I would go zipping along in the middle of Baltimore. Now, if you know the location of Johns Hopkins in Baltimore, you know that could be dangerous. I was prepared, though, with a sharp, pointed hammer in my hand at all times. When Dave Mirkin sponsored the two-mile "Run for Your Life," there I was at the starting line—my *first race!*

Perhaps, after seeing your friends enjoying the benefits of this sport, you have decided to have a go at it, too. As in any athletic endeavor, a beginner must start slowly. In fact, much of what you do at first is not running, but jogging.

"How do I know the difference?" people often ask.

According to Ken Cooper, nine minutes divides the two. (Others may suggest slightly varying amounts.) Can you complete a mile in nine minutes or less? If you can, you're running. If a mile takes you longer than nine minutes, you're jogging.

Running or jogging requires very little equipment— one reason it's so popular. A good pair of shoes, comfortable running clothes (shorts and a t-shirt for most of us), are all anyone needs. According to Arthur Lyiard, an Australian running trainer, shoes are over-designed for the majority of runners. Good shoes allow the foot to flow most normally on the ground. Insoles, arch supports and counters may be necessary to promote this in some cases. I happen to have a high arch so, for long runs of ten miles or more, I use an extremely high arch support. This removes undue pressure between the ball and heel of my foot, allowing me to run longer with the least possible strain.

The beginning runner should start by jogging at a slow pace, and only until tired. Form varies, but many experts advise that the pelvis should be tilted in slightly. Lean forward a little, too—to where you feel at ease—so you're not bouncing at the hips. Hands should be kept fairly low. Land on the ball of the foot; then roll to the back for short distance, the opposite for long distance later on.

There are three vital words to remember: do not push! Who knows how many aspiring runners ignore this advice and quit in discouragement? Perfectly outfitted in their ultimate air-cushioned running shoes and their monogrammed shorts with matching shirt, they turn out for the first day's workout. Checking their watches, with a quick glance around to see if anyone is looking, they are off and running at full speed.

Bad enough for someone already in good shape, this could be downright *dangerous* if you're out of condition. It takes time to attain a runner's physique and circulatory system. Muscles do not develop overnight. All of us remember overdoing something at one time or another in our lives, and the way we paid for it later. (Remember my ski trip to Jackson Hole?) Pride can raise its ugly head in even the most humble saint, but resist. Take it slow. Go easy. You'll discover your body adjusts quickly if you work out wisely.

Once you are able to jog slowly for a moderate distance, you can work your way up until you can jog comfortably for twenty to thirty minutes. Review Dr. Cooper's sound advice mentioned earlier: a total of twelve to fifteen miles per week, or four sessions of twenty to thirty minutes.

"Now, Ken, many of us run longer than that, because we have other goals in mind beside preventing heart disease," I reminded Ken Cooper one evening when we and our wives were out to dinner together. (He does my periodic physical exams, so he knows my exercise routine.) "We run because we *enjoy* it. Running gives us a feeling of well-being. We sleep better, and some of us, like me, just love to eat, so we run for weight control. I run to be a better competitor, even though I'm at the back of most races." The gist of his response was, "Well, it's O.K. if a person can do it, but exercise caution to prevent injury from overuse."

If you follow a sensible, systematic approach to running, pain will give way to strength, even joy. When this happens, you may want to consider developing a serious running program. Should this be the case, stop! Consult your doctor before going any further.

## Competitive Running

Maybe your exercise program will become so worthwhile that you'll want to expand into the realm of competition and longer distance. The same advice holds true. A complete physical exam is a must for anyone wanting to embark on such a strenuous regime. Go to your own doctor, or a physician of good repute, and tell him what you have in mind. Let him give you a thorough examination. Then, once he pronounces the go-ahead, get ready to start training for that first race.

Competition inspires me to push myself, not to beat others. If I didn't compete, I wouldn't be as disciplined, and I'd let myself drift. Races simply give me a goal to work toward. Are you the kind of person who likes something to aim at, too? It's safe to assume that your desire to compete includes a desire to improve. How about doing some timed intervals, for example? Set some distances and run them repeatedly within a specific time limit. They will help you increase speed, in addition to serving as a guide. Individual condition will determine the actual distance of the intervals; however, a good starting point is either quarter, half or one-mile runs. A brief resting period, consisting of walking and/or stretching, should fill the gap between runs.

Running can be habit-forming. With a few races under your belt, you may find yourself wishing to go even further, intrigued by the thought of that first marathon. Please don't be like me in my first marathon. I remember it well, in the beautiful southern Florida city of Ft. Myers. A friend had encouraged me to enter. "If you're running six-minute miles, Jim, you'll have no trouble doing a marathon," he assured me. So off I went. The race was on. I noticed I was leading the pack for the first ten miles and that ego boost really inspired me. The thought of *winning* my first marathon! Well, needless to say...I walked the last five miles. Nobody advised me to pace myself.

The ability to endure races of thirteen, twenty-six (marathon), fifty, one hundred or even two hundred miles comes from a base of long training runs. A person who does not occasionally run long in training will find it virtually impossible to compete in the ultra-distance runs. As the distance of these runs increases, so too should the time allotted for recovery. Cross-training becomes invaluable then because you can continue to keep active between runs.

Another word of caution: competitive runners often suffer from a variety of injuries. Among them are shin-splints (pain on the front of the leg from small tears in the leg muscles where they connect to the shin bone), illiotibial band friction syndrome (stinging pain usually felt on the outer part of the knee, caused by rubbing of the iliotibial band), stress fractures (cracks in the bone from excessive pounding), and muscle cramps. Moderation is the key to successful injury prevention. You can decrease risk even further by faithful stretching before, during and after running. In over a quarter-century of running, I have never had any serious injuries.

My own training schedule is relatively simple. I leave the house at about 5:00 a.m. and run twelve miles to work every day. Three days a week, Heather has started riding a bike along beside me. We talk and pray, or just be together. As we're moving along, we'll often exchange ideas about a favorite quote she has found in a book she's been reading.

In the evening when I get home, especially during the summer, I bike or swim for about half an hour. Sometimes I intersperse one or two days of interval or hill running, and other runs planned solely for pleasure that fit into my work and leisure schedule. During the weekend I complete my one long weekly run of about twenty miles.

My best advice? Learn to enjoy yourself while you run. Running with your spouse, friends or even your dog can greatly enhance those times out on the road. I prefer early morning because I feel as if I'm the master of my own schedule before anyone else at the clinic gets to it. Runners who set aside the first part of the day tend to be more consistent over the years.

For those of you who already are morning runners, are you tired of taking the same old route to work each day? Search out new ways to get to the office. Have fun! It will restore your enthusiasm and appreciation for life, even if only for the days you don't run.

## Walking Does Wonders

Walking has earned an excellent reputation as a healthy exercise for everyone, not just for older people. In fact, relative to the benefits it provides, Ken Cooper ranks walking among his top five preferred aerobic activities. It strengthens the heart and provides many of the same results as running, without the potential joint, bone and muscle injuries. One drawback to walking is the time involved. Walking takes longer to achieve the same training effect.

A big plus for this sport is the short and sweet list of required equipment: a pair of comfortable, but sturdy walking shoes. Just be sure the soles are thick enough to prevent bruising your feet. Running shoes will even work in place of the more expensive walking shoes on the market.

Walking is relatively easy on the body, but you should still start slowly. Work your way up to a speed that will carry you a distance of three miles in forty-five minutes, more than sufficient for beginners. If walking is your sole source of aerobic exercise, you should go on these three-mile jaunts four or five times each week. Enjoy the important social aspect of the sport; you'll be able to talk easily with a friend as you go. It does seem to make the time go faster.

There are several ways to increase the intensity and cut down the time factor in walking. First, you might try climbing an incline or steps while maintaining the same pace as over flat ground. Carry small weights, such as "Heavy Hands," to increase energy demand. They are relatively inexpensive, and are well worth the cost in minutes saved.

You can combine walking with any of the other aerobic exercises to create a well-rounded routine. Done this way, you multiply benefits and eliminate the danger of eventual boredom. Remember, too, even walkers require warm-up and cool-down periods.

## Weight Training Works

You can enhance the value of aerobic exercise by using weights to strengthen and tone specific muscle groups. Working out with weights is *anaerobic*, not a cardiovascular conditioner like aerobics, so you need both kinds of exercise "Why would I need stronger muscles?" women often wonder. Think of household tasks that require lifting, or carrying young children. Wouldn't those duties be much easier if a woman were stronger? She reduces the chance of straining muscles or collapsing from exhaustion at the end of the day.

As a unique individual, you have your own goals and requirements. Therefore, a good program will be tailored to meet your personal needs. Generally, light to medium weights are suitable for all but the serious weight lifter. They will increase muscle tone and provide moderate strength increases without decreasing muscle flexibility (stretching capacity). That commodity is too valuable to be sacrificed for bulk and strength derived from heavy weight lifting.

While you can purchase inexpensive weights and train at home, many experts recommend otherwise. If you begin a program in a gym or health club, a professional can assist you in developing a routine for your specific needs and then monitor you for proper form. At a fitness center you often have access to Nautilus equipment, some of the most effective available. Nautilus training makes the best use of both time and effort.

Long or intense workouts should be limited to no more than three times a week. Muscles need time to recover from the tearing down that occurs during the training session. A rest day prevents stiffness also. If weight training becomes so enjoyable that you wish to exercise every day, simply alternate specific muscle groups; work the upper body one day and the lower body the next. Remember that weight training is in *addition* to aerobic exercise, not a substitute for it.

## The Massage Message

*Ouch!* We've probably all endured the pain and stiffness of a hypertonic (very rigid) muscle. *Ahhh* . . . a properly trained and licensed therapist can, by applying varying degrees of pressure through a combination of strokes and manipulations, relieve the stiffness in the affected muscle and connective tissue. Result: the natural neuromuscular balance returns.

Athletes of all ages and sports use massage. Done properly, it relaxes muscles, stimulates blood flow and releases areas of tightness and tension. Jan Gallahue, a massage therapist from Clearwater, Florida, supplied information for this brief overview of massage.

The enhanced circulation produced by massage increases the flow of energy to the muscles and quickly removes any fatigue-causing waste materials from the tissues. As a result, the rate of recovery increases. Fatigue will diminish more rapidly, injuries will occur less often and when they do, they will heal more quickly. Then the athlete can resume training.

Stress, caused by over-exertion, injury and poor posture results in tension. This tension can lead to a loss of appetite, insomnia and despondency, all of which interfere with the wellness of the body, mind and spirit. Consequently, a growing number of people from all walks of life have begun seeking relief from pain and stress at the hands of massage therapists. With this has come an increase in their own self-awareness and a heightened sense of well-being.

Use caution when choosing a massage therapist. The safest way to locate one of good-repute is by personal referral. Check with massage schools or health clubs in your area who might offer massage as one of their services. Also, some therapeutic clinics provide massage therapy in addition to chiropractic care.

## For Senior Citizens Only

I am partial to seniors, as most of St. Luke's patients fall in this age group. To see them stay healthier, longer, is one of my fondest desires. Wise use of exercise among the elderly may be one of the best medicines available. As the body ages, it tends to lose muscle mass and gain fat tissue. After the age of twenty-five, muscle tissue reduction occurs at about one-half per cent per year and fat increases at one per cent per year. This statistic is not etched in stone, though. You can alter it through a system of constant conditioning.

Dr. Gabe Mirkin, nationally-known fitness expert, in his book, *Getting Thin,* states,

> It is true that almost all of us will reach the point where we can no longer exercise as well as we once did....The encroachment is slow and gradual, but most of us can notice its effects by the time we reach forty.
>
> Nevertheless, we do have a say in slowing the aging process somewhat. By exercising and eating properly, we can retain most of our fitness through our fifties and sixties, and even beyond. At the age of eighty, artist Norman Rockwell was still riding a bicycle five miles every day.[2]

If Norman Rockwell could do it, so can you. According to the Tampa Tribune, the University of Florida's Center for Exercise Science in Gainesville proved in a recent study that exercise benefits the elderly. Forty-nine untrained people, aged seventy to seventy-nine (in good health), participated in the twenty-four week study.

They began working out three times a week in one of two areas: weight training on Nautilus equipment or endurance training through walking and jogging. Individuals in both groups lost weight, about two and a quarter pounds of fat and just under an inch in waist size, stated physiologist James Graves. Those who did endurance work increased endurance, but not strength; likewise, people who worked on strengthening improved strength, but not endurance. Since both strength *and* endurance are necessary, the study shows that a well-balanced routine is just as important for seniors.

A fitness program adapted to meet your special needs can help slow the aging process. Your attitude about life will improve and you will look, feel and act younger. Age has never been a barrier to fitness. Look at Caleb, that Old Testament hero of faith. At the tender age of eighty-five, he began the conquest of the mountain he inherited in the promised land. In his own words he gives testimony to the virtues of conditioning,

> *"And now behold, I am eighty-five years old today. I am still as strong today as I was in the day Moses sent me; as my strength was then, so my strength is now, for war and for going out and coming in. Now then, give me this hill country about which the Lord spoke on that day, for you heard on that day that Anakim were there, with great fortified cities; perhaps the Lord will be with me, and I shall drive them out as the Lord has spoken."*
>
> Joshua 14:10b-12a

That Caleb was a "go-getter," wasn't he? Although you probably don't have any giant Anakim to chase out of walled cities (in the physical realm, anyway), you can still stay in shape. All the aerobic activities mentioned thus far are open to those in their seventies, eighties and nineties. Admittedly, it will require discipline and commitment, but the rewards are well worth the effort. Start s-l-o-w-l-y! My previous recommendation applies especially to you. Begin with a brisk walk, light calisthenics, swimming or biking. Consider starting the day off with your exercise program. You will elevate your body to a higher metabolic rate, preparing you to meet the needs of daily living.

Why not share your exercise routine with others and make it more enjoyable for them and you? By giving yourself to help meet the needs of another person, you may be doing yourself the greatest service. In giving, you receive.

## Choosing a Good Fitness Center

*Your personal commitment* is the primary ingredient. Then look for the following criteria: a professionally-trained director and staff who practice what they preach, a broad spectrum of health services, the latest in well-maintained equipment and facilities, individualized instruction and group activities, a clean, pleasant atmosphere and helpful attitude, good hours and reasonable fees.

Total Fitness Center in Tarpon Springs, Florida serves as an excellent example of a non-hospital based wellness center. President and Director, Dean Cosgrove, is a Double Iron Man competitor, holds a master's degree in exercise science and a doctorate in health sciences. Many staff members hold related degrees, as well. Services for a total wellness lifestyle at TFC include extensive testing, Cardiac Rehabilitation, Medical Weight Management, Physical Therapy, and Arthritis Aquatic Therapy. Numerous options in weight machines, bicycles, and treadmills, racquetball courts, pool, plus amenities complete the fitness picture.

# 4. The Eating-For-Life Diet

**"I**t sounds like a 'gag-me' diet, but it was a good plan," pastor and best-selling author Chuck Swindoll commented lightheartedly on one of his radio broadcasts. He was referring to the famous Old Testament prophet, Daniel, and his strict dietary regimen. You may remember the account of the young Hebrew who was chosen to serve in the courts of the Babylonian king, Nebuchadnezzar.

*"But Daniel made up his mind that he would not defile himself with the king's choice food or with the wine which he drank; so he sought permission from the commander of the officials that he might not defile himself"* (Daniel 1:8). He proposed that his simple diet of vegetables would work better than the king's choicest sweetmeats. It did, too, for Daniel and the others who were diligent with him. After ten days they all looked healthier than the youths who were eating the king's rich foods. America, a nation of overweight people perpetually "on a diet," can learn from Daniel and his friends.

"I can't seem to cope with even the basic problems of life," complain many of Dr. Ray Wunderlich's patients. He has found that in case after case, a change in dietary habits transforms his patients' outlook on life. And what a transformation! No longer forced to merely react to outward circumstances, they now recognize a wide range of options.

After years of experience in his field, Dr. Wunderlich has collected viable evidence that good nutrition can revitalize anyone mentally, and help him or her make the right choices for healthy living. He believes that everything you do—finding a job and keeping it, choosing a life partner in marriage, handling stressful situations, or simply dealing with people, will be much easier when a proper diet fuels the activity.

Unfortunately, the Standard American Diet is SAD, indeed. In the 1988 report on nutrition and disease, Surgeon General C. Everett Koop warned that improper diet is associated with five of the ten leading causes of death in this country. Many preventive-oriented physicians have seen firsthand evidence of poor health induced by the SAD diet. Excessively high in salt, fat, calories, protein, refined sugar, chemical additives and processed foods, it drastically affects all the body systems. Not only does physical health suffer from a poor diet; reactions to life's situations are affected, as well.

It's no use trying to live under a blanket of ignorance, attempting to support an illusion of invincibility. "You are what you eat," as the saying goes. The word behavior, in its broadest meaning encompasses thoughts that enter the mind as well as physical actions. Dr. Wunderlich cites several examples of how diet can affect behavior.

Chocolate, he says, contains the same chemical (phenylethylamine) associated with the emotion of love—hence the popular craving for that sweet, brown stuff. Criminals, both juvenile and adult, consume an unusually high number of soft drinks and milk products. Men who are spouse-abusers tend to consume huge quantities of meat. Now, this does not imply that if you like meat you will abuse your wife, or if you enjoy drinking soda you will wind up looking out from behind prison bars. It simply means that you should use wisdom and moderation in planning your diet because it does affect your behavior and attitudes.

## When and How Often To Eat?

A nutritionally balanced diet requires more than knowing what food to eat and what to avoid. *Timing* of meals remains a topic of wide discussion among expert nutritionists. One side adheres to "healthful snacking" intermittently throughout the day. The other group supports the theory that all eating should be limited to two or three regular meals. Each side gives supporting evidence and both are worth investigating.

Regular meals are the keystone of proper diet. Many experts advise trying to establish a rhythm of eating. It matters not whether you eat two or three meals, as long as you do it at an expected time. The sun rises and sets with dependability; so, too, is the body a creature of habit. Establishing regularity of meals lets the body rest.

When you eat substantial meals without snacking in between, you enhance your health, according to Dr. Wunderlich. Each time you eat, your pancreas releases insulin into the blood stream. Frequent and prolonged exposure of the arteries to simple sugars, cholesterol and insulin may favor the development of fatty deposits on the arterial walls. This condition, known as atherosclerosis, may lead to heart attacks, strokes and many other complications. Long rest periods between meals permit fat build-ups to clear out of the bloodstream.

Dr. Gabe Mirkin supports the theory of "healthful snacking." Brown fat, a minute amount whose sole purpose is heating the body's vital organs, receives energy to perform its task from calories consumed. A greater overall caloric burn-off results when brown fat keeps working hard during the day. According to Dr. Mirkin, this can best be accomplished by continually ingesting calories in smaller, more frequent meals. In **Getting Thin,** his exceptional book on fat and weight loss, he advises patients to eat five or six small meals throughout the day. The key: be careful not to exceed the recommended caloric intake, as it affects the function of "brown fat."

How many times have you gotten up late for work or school and been forced to skip breakfast? Can you recall feeling especially tired and weak early in the day? Dizzy, even faint? This is not unusual. These symptoms often result from low blood sugar (glucose), a chemical which helps the brain function efficiently. Eating breakfast serves to replenish the supply of glucose stored in the liver, but the meal must be high in complex carbohydrates. Never sacrifice breakfast, if you can avoid it. Experts from both sides readily agree upon the importance of a high-complex-carbohydrate, high-fiber start to the day.

## Making Calories Your Friends, Not Enemies

"Wednesday Special: Barbecued Pork Ribs—All U Can Eat—$3.99." Restaurants use drawing cards like this to lure passers-by to sample their wares. How many of us can really afford to eat *all* we want and not worry about the consequences? Not many, I dare say. There are, however, exceptions to every rule. Among every gathering of people, you can find at least one person who can devour mountains of food without gaining a single pound. Strawberry shortcake, hot fudge sundaes, sirloin tips and lobster bisque. And they stay thin.

My secretary, Anne, fits this description, if anyone ever did. She's thirty-six years old, 5'7" tall, weighs a hundred twelve pounds and eats "all the time," in her own words. Does she concern herself with the types of foods she eats? No, not very often. There's always a Danish roll or a big chocolate brownie on her desk. If you are like Anne, you may be tempted to skip the rest of this section, but I ask you to resist the urge (you too, Anne!). Changes that may not yet be apparent in blood tests could already be taking place on the inside.

People burn calories at different rates, as I'm sure you have noticed by now. A hyperactive person possesses a low percentage of body fat, and will burn more carbohydrates, protein and fat than someone living a sedentary life. Let both eat the same amount of calories and the slower-moving person will gain more fat than his energetic counterpart.

Endocrine changes can occur in the body and cause foods and fluids to be absorbed at a faster rate, leading to abnormal weight gain. Although researchers consider this another of life's inequalities, they agree that practically anyone who did not receive a metabolically efficient body at birth can develop one through proper diet and exercise.

Would you like to be the contented owner of a healthy temple? Such an aspiration requires your supply of calories to be perfectly matched to your body's demand for them. Diet and exercise can be so coordinated that every calorie goes toward providing for the needs of your body.

You may recall how the gas wars of years gone by drove the price of gasoline to rock bottom. That was a case where the consumer reaped the benefits of an abundant fuel supply. Consume too much body fuel in calories, however, and you will surely reap the *"unbenefits"*... obesity.

No matter how you look at it, a calorie is a calorie is a calorie. Every calorie above the required base amount increases your chances of gaining weight and raising your cholesterol level. As you have already read, a balanced diet and regular exercise together can help build a healthy temple. Approximately twenty-five per cent of caloric intake is expended through exertion. The remaining seventy-five per cent goes to fuel basal metabolism, the rate the body burns calories while resting. Everybody's basal metabolism predisposes them to be either fat or skinny. Knowing this, you can lose or gain weight as needed.

On the average, a daily intake of 2400 calories is adequate to sustain a middle-aged man of one hundred fifty-five pounds, while a middle-aged woman at her ideal weight of one hundred twenty pounds requires about 1800 calories. These figures may vary from one individual to another because of the body's natural efficiency.

Frank Shorter, a former world-class marathoner, points out that the body does not need even that much fuel. He feels a base of 1200-1500 calories will suffice. The body becomes more effective at lower-than-normal caloric levels.

No one meal should contain more than forty per cent of your total daily calorie consumption. Spread those calories evenly throughout the day, whether you eat two or three larger meals or several smaller ones. Remember that most experts agree on the following point: it's best not to eat within two hours of bedtime.

There is more to a balanced diet than deciding when to eat. *What* to eat is another question. Properly balanced, a good diet mainly consists of complex carbohydrates (vegetables and grains), protein (broiled fish, lean meats, skinned chicken) and fat (peanut butter and vegetable oils).

At the University of South Florida College of Medicine, Division of Cardiology, Dr. Knight and his colleagues have gathered scientific data about diet for a healthy heart and body. Add fiber, reduce sodium, keep protein to a maximum of twenty to forty grams a day, and all fats at thirty per cent of total caloric intake (ten per cent of that amount in saturated fats). Enjoy a liberal use of whole grains, pasta, fruit, rice, potatoes, fresh vegetables, any type of bran, fish (especially the deep-water oily variety), and natural fish oil supplements.

Dr. Knight follows closely the American Heart Association guidelines and those of The National Research Council (NRC), an arm of the National Academy of Sciences. The NRC released a 1300-page report in 1989 about diet and health that suggests *complex carbohydrates* at a level of *fifty-five per cent* or more and *fat* at *thirty per cent* or less of total calories. In other words, if your daily calorie allowance is 1500, then at least 825 calories should consist of whole grains, fruits and vegetables. Fat should comprise no more than 450 calories for the day.

So much for agreement. Dr. Nathan Pritikin's diet, very low in protein, fat, cholesterol, salt, and high in fiber, is at the far end of the spectrum. His stringent advice suggests the following ratio: *eighty per cent* of total calories from *complex carbohydrates, ten per cent protein* and *ten per cent fat.* On a 1500 calorie-a-day diet, that would mean 1200 calories from carbohydrates, 150 from protein, and 150 from fat (for example, four ounces of skinned, broiled chicken and four teaspoons of vegetable oil per day).

I have found it to be simple and sensible. Some people, like L.A. pathologist and runner Dr. Tom Bassler, argue that marathon runners should not be so restricted. For me, it works well.

Even if you're pressed for time, the Pritikin program makes a way for you to eat right. Their pre-cooked dinners are now available in simple microwave-safe containers and can be ordered from California for about four dollars each. They are reasonably tasty and provide all the necessary calories so you won't have to do any calculating. Following the strict Pritikin diet consistently takes a little self-discipline, but it's worth the commitment.

Prior to the Pritikin regime, the rice diet at Duke University showed near-miraculous cures for people with diabetes, high blood pressure and many other diseases. It called for limited protein and high amounts of complex carbohydrates from rice. The problem was that very few people could continue to eat that way, largely because of so little variety.

If you would like to stay healthy, build your diet around nutritious foods. Nature's foods. In summary, concentrate on eating vegetables and beans, whole grains, lean meats, skimmed dairy products and polyunsaturated fats. Avoid sugars, saturated fats, white flour, chemical additives and the snacks that contain them. Everyone would do well to eliminate margarine and butter from their diet.

Your body requires carbohydrates for a ready fuel supply, especially if you're getting plenty of exercise. Unfortunately, in our society, simple carbohydrates from sweetened cold drinks and sodas, candy, cookies, donuts, buns and white breads replace the right kind from fresh fruits, vegetables and grains. Feel free to eliminate all of the former gooey, fattening group.

Who hasn't heard of a "steak and potatoes man?" He prides himself on being the image of a normal, run-of-the-mill, plain and simple kind of guy. The plain and simple lifestyle may be a thing of the past for many Americans in all but one respect—diet. They'd do better to drop the steak and leave the plain potatoes. Too much protein from animal products (more of a realistic danger here in the U.S. than a protein deficiency) produces mineral loss in the body and promotes degenerative diseases.

## More Truth About Fat and Cholesterol

Fats are a potentially serious trouble spot. Some Americans derive almost half of their calories from fats—butter, margarine, fried foods, snack foods, and desserts. (That might be why The National Research Council thought they would do well to recommend thirty per cent.) Usually, adequate protein supplies needed fat in the diet.

Remember those people like my secretary who eat all they want and never gain an ounce? They *may* beat the odds in cholesterol, too. During the recent "wellness days" we sponsored for St. Luke's staff, coordinator and triathlete Cheryl Durstein-Decker told Anne she had one of the lowest cholesterol levels she had ever seen among mid-thirty year-olds: 129. My response when I found out . . . "This just isn't fair!" (Actually, a level too low may not be ideal, either.)

Most people must avoid fats high in cholesterol. You can spot these easily because they remain solid at room temperature and are mostly dairy or animal fat. Try using one dietician's yardstick: if a food grows in the ground, it contains no cholesterol. The margarine vs. butter war still rages. Some studies suggest that the introduction of margarine has brought a parallel in the increase of cardiovascular disease, so it may be more dangerous than butter. If you insist on margarine, the liquid form is probably better than solid. Better yet, try to develop a taste for food without it. Your heart and blood vessels will love you more each day.

Look for other fats that are liquid at room temperature, especially the polyunsaturated kind found in soybeans, walnut, and linseed oils or fish. For certain high cholesterol diseases, polyunsaturated fats may even be therapeutic. Here's a handy "fat fact": fifteen grams of marine fat a day at nine calories per gram equal 135 calories. That's more than a ten per cent fat allowance on a 1200 calorie diet, so there would be no room left for butter, margarine, or other fats.

Ken Cooper has written a highly informative, new book entitled, *Controlling Cholesterol.* Since the subject has grown enough to fill an entire 350-page book, our discussion here will barely scratch the surface. With all the publicity geared towards lowering cholesterol levels, you may be surprised to learn its vital function in the body. A forerunner to all steroid hormones, cholesterol plays a part in both absorption of fats by the intestines and conversion of the sun's ultraviolet rays to vitamin D.

Large concentrations of this waxy substance reside in the brain and nerve tissues. Cholesterol is distributed throughout the body, as well. Although you need cholesterol, it's not necessary to consume it. The body, God's miracle of creation, supplies an adequate amount, mainly from the liver.

Cholesterol always moves about in the bloodstream with an "escort," called lipoprotein, either low-density (LDL) or high-density lipoprotein (HDL). LDL deposits cholesterol on the walls of the blood vessels. Left unattended, cholesterol continues to collect, forming atherosclerotic plaque. There it can restrict, and even completely block, the flow of blood. End result...stroke or heart attack.

In God's infinite wisdom, He prepared for this eventuality. He did not leave you defenseless; He created beneficial HDL, high-density lipoprotein. HDL picks up the deposits of cholesterol left by LDL and carries them to the gall bladder, where the potentially deadly build-ups are converted to bile acids, aiding digestion. A thorough physical exam will determine actual HDL and LDL levels. Ideally, low-density lipoprotein levels should be low while high-density lipoprotein should be high.

Thus, you can see the reasons for the dietary goals mentioned earlier: add polyunsaturated fats such as fatty fish and fish oils to increase beneficial HDL levels. At the same time, refrain from eating animal fats that increase harmful LDL levels.

The Pritikin diet is excellent for people who need therapeutic treatment for high cholesterol, as well as for those who simply want to stay in peak physical condition. For example, one year at the Ironman competition in Hawaii, seven out of the top ten finishers were on the Pritikin diet.

Strenuous exercise also has a positive affect on cholesterol in the body. For example, my total cholesterol/HDL ratio can get down as low as two-to-one after five months of intensive training for the Double Ironman. When I ease off after the event, it returns to my normal three-to-one ratio within a short time.

New research steadily emerges which points to a substance other than animal fat as the prime culprit in LDL increases. Consequently, it unveils this chemical as a leading cause of heart attack. Dr. Linus Pauling has considerable insight into this controversial area.

In his informative book, *How to Live Longer and Feel Better,* Dr. Pauling refers to a study in Framingham, Massachusetts. Conducted under the auspices of the National Institute of Health, the research shows that limiting intake of cholesterol by decreasing eggs and animal fat does not necessarily reduce the cholesterol level in the blood. Subsequently, neither would increasing the amounts consumed raise that level because the body manufactures cholesterol in its cells daily. Production automatically decreases when the dietary intake increases, and vice versa.

What else, then, causes cholesterol to increase in those who have coronary disease? For an answer, Dr. Pauling points to studies done by John Yudkin and Milton Winitz. Yudkin noticed that coronary disease patients ate more sucrose, or white sugar, than those without heart trouble. For six months, Yudkin and Winitz observed eighteen institution-alized adults who were fed strictly-monitored food. They had no access to any dietary supplements. Over the course of the experiment their diet was changed several times, with dramatic results.

For the first four weeks the subjects were fed a balanced diet of essential amino acids (protein), vitamins, minerals, complex carbohydrates and a small amount of fat. After only two weeks the average blood cholesterol level dropped from 227 milligrams per deciliter to 173 milligrams. Another two weeks passed and it had dropped even lower, to 160 milligrams. (A reading of 160 mg/dl or less is considered a good, safe amount.)

At this point the diet was changed, but only in one area. Refined sugar was substituted for one quarter of the complex carbohydrates. Almost immediately, blood cholesterol began to rise. Within one week it had climbed from 160 to 178. Then, two weeks later it was 208.

Rather than stop with this bit of information, the researchers went a step further and changed the diet one more time. Refined sugar was eliminated again and complex carbohydrates were added. By the end of a week, with the original test diet restored, the average level of blood cholesterol dropped to 175 and finally leveled off at 150 milligrams per deciliter. Dr. Pauling sees this as conclusive evidence that increased sugar in the diet causes an increase in cholesterol level. He presents a convincing argument that sugar consumption promotes heart disease.

Please don't use this study to justify adding more animal fat to the "approved foods" portion of your menu. On the contrary, fat is fat. You'll still do best to restrict it, whether it raises cholesterol levels or not. Rather than suddenly trying to cut out sugar altogether, begin by *reducing* your intake. You might be surprised to know that you should be wary of eating too many sweet fruits, as well. I noticed a tremendous increase in my cholesterol level during a period when I was eating large quantities of fruit (at least 1000 calories, more than ten servings a day). As soon as I cut back, my cholesterol level returned to normal.

Dr. Linus Pauling has one more tip for lowering your blood cholesterol level: take vitamin C. A high intake of vitamin C increases the rate at which cholesterol is removed from the blood and converted into bile acids. This process requires ascorbate, another name for vitamin C. Thus, a high amount of C reduces total cholesterol, especially dangerous LDL. As such, it restores the proper high/low ratio between HDL and LDL, and helps protect against heart attack.

## Nutritional Supplements— Should You or Not?

Mention vitamin and mineral supplements to a group of professionals and you will invariably invoke a wide variety of opinions. Dr. Wunderlich, provides his patients with a no-nonsense approach in his orientation manual. It reads,

> Your need for nutritional supplements is determined by history, physical examination, laboratory tests, how you feel, what you believe and how you react. Needs vary with each individual and may change over time with your body and dietary changes. Optimally, your nutrients should be supplied by your diet—with as few as possible supplements required. If you feel you have a need, buy them in small quantities until you are sure you have a continuing need for them and are tolerating them well. Some persons can take all their supplements at one time without a problem, while others must take them one at a time until they build their tolerance to them. As an example, supplements containing niacin may cause flushing, warmth, redness and itching. Many reactions usually diminish as succeeding doses are taken, and sometimes taking the supplement with meals or lowering the dose may provide relief.

Dr. Mirkin takes a similar cautionary approach. Not everyone needs supplements, he says, because vitamins last a long time in the body and are easily replaced when depleted. The recommended daily amounts cited by the National Academy of Sciences are readily available in the diets of most people. Only so much of a particular vitamin is needed to perform its function. Anything beyond that the body disposes of as waste.

If you feel you are lacking in vitamins, Dr. Mirkin suggests that you limit yourself to a daily multiple vitamin pill. Such a dosage should not cause any of the problems associated with extremely high vitamin intake. Examples? Too much vitamin A can cause joint pain and bone deterioration, while too much vitamin D can promote calcification of both the arteries and muscles. Massive doses of Vitamin C can trigger kidney stones and cause kidney damage. Too much vitamin B-3, or niacin, can cause liver damage and ulcers. Excessive vitamin E also causes liver damage, high blood pressure and blood clots. Mirkin recommends a mineral supplement of iron only during childbearing years, and calcium after menopause, if a woman is generally healthy.

Linus Pauling, on the other hand, has a contrary opinion. He sees vitamins as a buffer against disease. As such, they are a prime factor in preventive health. His reasons are thoroughly outlined in his book mentioned earlier, ***How to Live Longer and Feel Better.*** Briefly, his daily regimen of supplements is simple, but complete. He takes four tablets each evening: one 800 IU vitamin E capsule, Super B (B-vitamin complex) tablet, one vitamin-mineral tablet and one 25,000 IU vitamin A capsule. Before breakfast, he takes most of his vitamin C. In either orange juice or water, he dissolves three level teaspoons of pure crystalline ascorbic acid. He may add a little baking soda to make an effervescent drink. Sodium ascorbate can be substituted as a viable source of vitamin C.

As of April, 1989, Dr. Pauling's recipe of four tablets and eighteen grams of vitamin C (L-ascorbic acid, fine crystals) cost about fifty cents per day. You should work up gradually to such high doses of vitamins and minerals. (For more information, write: Bronson Pharmaceuticals, 4526 Rinetti Lane, La Canada, California 91011. Their toll-free number is 1-800-521-3322, or 1-800-521-3323 in California.) They are one of the most reasonably-priced sources I have found.

While all of these men are credible experts in their respective fields, you should discuss any personal deficiencies with a physician who specializes in nutrition. Let him perform various blood and urine tests to determine what you lack, if anything. He can then prescribe what you need to regain your vitamin and mineral balance.

Speaking of supplements, let me share a personal experience to bring a little levity to this ponderous subject. It was my very first Boston Marathon, back in 1971. In preparation for this esteemed event, I tried to be so careful to do everything right.

I heard that a marathoner needs high amounts of calcium and magnesium due to excretion in perspiration during the race. Since calcium acts as nature's muscle relaxer and helps prevent cramping, I wanted to be sure to avoid depletion. Have you ever heard that "more is better?" Believe me, it's not always true of supplements. I ate ten dolomite mineral tablets right before the race and had to stop for thirteen nature breaks along the way. Needless to say, my race time slowed down considerably.

## Nutrition for the Athlete

Optimal diet goes hand in hand with physical activity, for several reasons. Regular exercise actually increases the efficiency with which the body uses vitamins and minerals without increasing the need for them. It also raises the body's caloric need and helps regulate appetite. In fact, persons who exercise have been shown to eat less than their inactive counterparts.

Myths abound in every field of human endeavor; an athlete's diet is no exception. Some of the more popular misconceptions are as follows: "Vitamin supplements help athletes use more energy." "Athletes need protein for extra energy." "Protein builds bigger and stronger muscles."

Contrary to popular belief, the physically active person has no greater need for protein or fat than an inactive person. The high protein fad diets touted in the past produced more harmful effects than they did good. Protein makes an insignificant contribution to energy during exercise; therefore, maintaining it at a level of ten per cent of total caloric intake (Pritikin) is sufficient for the active person. Eat too much protein and you run the risk of mineral imbalance, loss of needed calcium through the urine, elevated blood cholesterol, fatigue, nausea, kidney malfunction, constipation and rapid weight gain after diet cessation.

Even for the athlete, fat should not exceed the recommended ten to thirty per cent of the daily caloric intake. Less is preferable because the body doesn't need dietary fat to maintain its fat stores. Any extra calories will be converted and stored as fat no matter what their source. Be careful to not *totally* eliminate fat from your diet because you could develop a deficiency of fatty acids, your heart's main source of energy. Most polyunsaturated fat sources, especially soybeans, walnuts, linseed and chestnuts are rich in fatty acids. If your fat intake ever falls below ten per cent, cardiac arrest could occur.

The preferred, critical energy source is complex carbohydrates. Sports require quick bursts of energy, so for an athlete to compete successfully, at least seventy percent of daily calories should fall within this food group. The greater majority should be complex (grains, starchy vegetables), as opposed to simple sugars (fruits and sweets). Complex carbohydrates provide needed fiber, vitamins and minerals. They take longer to digest and keep you feeling full, longer.

Carbohydrates, when metabolized, become glycogen, which provides a ready fuel for those immediate muscle actions so common to sports. Glycogen also helps maintain normal blood sugar levels while you are resting or sleeping.

Fatigue, dehydration and energy loss are symptoms of low carbohydrate intake, as evidenced by a lack of the presence of glycogen. If you are an athlete battling the above symptoms, try increasing complex carbohydrates.

Nutritional habits before and during competition vary from one individual to another. Some prepare for a race by "carbohydrate overloading," eating small meals of vegetables, breads and pastas for two or three days prior to the event. This builds reserves of glycogen, which is particularly important in races of marathon length or longer. Yet, all overloading techniques aside, many runners feel best with an empty stomach at race time. I prefer not to eat heavy foods twelve to eighteen hours before a marathon.

Some athletes drink fluids containing caffeine and sugar in preparation. I drink sugared tea two hours before the race, and again fifteen minutes right beforehand. During the actual run, fluids high in electrolytes and sugar (like Gatorade) keep me hydrated and energized. Over the years, I have learned that this combination works best for me.

"Water consumed during exercise can cause cramping," is a popular rumor which could not be further from the truth. Water is necessary, particularly during long periods of exercise, like marathons, when the body runs the risk of dehydration. Before a prolonged workout I drink more water than I actually need. I prefer it cold—refrigerator temperature—because the body absorbs cold water faster, aiding hydration and minimizing the discomfort of a full stomach.

## Senior Citizens' Diet Special

As I mentioned, you seniors are a select group. To feel your best, you require an appropriate diet and supplements. Keep simplicity in mind as the ideal. Your personal physician has no doubt already made dietary suggestions to you. If you take his advice, you could avoid an ultimatum from him later on.

Remember that with age, the tendency to gain fat increases—about one per cent per year after age twenty-five. It can be dealt with through a combination of diet and exercise. Your need for calories will only decrease if your activity level decreases.

Of course, you would do well to avoid caffeine, nicotine, white sugar and white flour. If your blood pressure tends to be high, limit your use of sodium (salt) and the foods containing it. Concentrate more on raw vegetables that are so good for you and be sure all fat has been trimmed from any meat. Cut down on those other fatty foods which clog your blood vessels.

Eat your food throughout the day in quantities as small as possible. This way, you avoid over-taxing your digestive system. It has already been working hard for quite a few years. Remember, too, the least amount you can eat is probably best. You might even keep a record of your eating habits. Charting these and any changes that occur can be invaluable as you adjust your diet for better health.

## Final Food Thoughts

Once you know the foods your body needs to stay healthy, you must seek a supply source. Supermarkets are becoming more in tune with the public outcry for nutritious choices. Roadside stands and health food stores are also good places. No matter where you choose to shop be an avid label reader (even at the local health food store). Know the ingredients in the food you buy.

Having carefully selected and prepared your food, learn to chew it thoroughly. Also, try to avoid large quantities of liquids with your meals, This helps prevent overeating, one unfortunate by-product of an abundant food supply. Behind every cupboard lingers the tendency to eat, just because it's there. Should you ever spot this fault, shift your attention to more meaningful activities.

Have you come to the conclusion that your dietary habits are in need of *drastic* change? If so, guard against discouragement. Don't set yourself up for failure by trying to change everything overnight. You can build long-lasting, healthy habits more easily through making specific, short-term improvements. To help you get started, follow these basic guidelines Dr. Wunderlich uses to encourage his patients.

Begin with candy bars. Your first goal should be to reduce them by fifty per cent. Once you accomplish this, move on to soft drinks and do the same thing. After you have successfully met these two goals, tackle salt and do the same. From there, move on to fat and then to meats. Do not try to cut out all these things at once, but work on one area at a time (unless the substance is life-threatening, of course). Your final goal should be to increase the amount of vegetables, fruits, whole grains and fish by fifty per cent. For me, filling up on vegetable juice, like V-8, satisfies hunger, adds vitamins and minerals and helps me avoid the urge to drink sugary beverages.

| Reduce by 50% | Increase by 50% |
|---|---|
| candy | vegetables |
| soft drinks | whole grains |
| salt | fruits |
| fat | fish |
| meat | |

You can gain helpful encouragement and assistance in developing healthy new habits by seeking knowledgeable professionals in the field of nutrition. Look first for those who have successfully made such changes themselves. Begin with your regular physician, local hospitals, mental health clinics and health agencies. Even the media is a good starting point. You can find the necessary information and support to help improve your chances of a long, active life, once you embrace the desire to change.

As we close this section on maintaining the outer court of your temple—your body—I'd like to quote from the foreward to Dr. Mary Ruth Swope's book, ***Are You Sick and Tired of Feeling Sick and Tired?,*** which was written by a friend of mine, pastor and author Jamie Buckingham:

> Last year, after being 50 pounds overweight for half of my life, I realized I was dying. I had watched some of my friends die for some of the same reasons I was dying, and I determined that age 50 was not God's time for me to go to heaven—or wherever else fat people go when they eat themselves to death.
>
> I also realized that simply desiring to be healthy would not get the job done. I had wanted to be healthy ever since I got fat. But each day brought the same results. Defeat.
>
> Gradually I became aware that it takes more than desire—it takes commitment. Not just commitment to lose weight—but a commitment to change your lifestyle in regard to nutrition, exercise, and image.
>
> The results were dramatic. And have been lasting. By proper eating and exercise I dropped from 225 pounds to 165—and there I shall stay the rest of my life....
>
> Remember, it takes more than desire. It takes commitment. But once you've tasted life, you'll never want to go back to the way of death.[3]

To that, I say "Amen!"

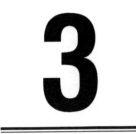

# 3

# LIFE IN THE HOLY PLACE: YOUR MIND

# 5. Potential Unlimited?

Plunge to the depths of the seas. Soar to the fringes of the universe. Explore the intricacies of the atom. Caress the velvety softness of a baby's skin. Grieve over the loss of a loved one. All are born of the vast resources of the mind, with capabilities yet unfathomed. Thought. Reason. Memory. Personality. Emotions. Will. These are just a few of the innumerable attributes of your mind and the activities it performs every day.

"Soul" is another biblical name for this part of your being, so I will use "mind" and "soul" interchangeably. According to Webster's Unabridged Dictionary, the mind comprises, "(a) that which thinks, perceives, feels, wills, etc.; seat or subject of consciousness; (b) the thinking and perceiving part of consciousness; intellect or intelligence; (c) all of an individual's conscious experiences; (d) the conscious and the unconscious together as a unit, psyche..."[1]

The organ or seat of the mind, of course, is the brain. In the *Reader's Digest* best-selling book, ***I Am Joe's Body*** by J.D. Ratcliff, Joe's brain proudly shares a physiological self-description. He minces no words in telling the reader what an amazing organ he is. Scientists know relatively little about him, he says, compared to his extraordinary qualifications. Other miracles of creation can't quite measure up to his capabilities. They're enough to befuddle the latest state-of-the-art computer, even though he weighs in at only about three pounds. He's not much to look at, either—just a lump of gray and white matter resembling gelatin with wrinkles. Appearances certainly are deceiving, aren't they?

Joe's brain goes on to set the record straight. The wonderful senses of touch, sight and hearing Joe enjoys are actually the brain's doing, not the fingers, eyes and ears. Of course, his brain proves right. Although the eye particularly fascinates me (I've specialized in ophthalmology all these years), I have to agree that the miracle of sight would fall short without the brain. It contains a veritable treasure chest of a person's lifelong memories. In fact, to hear Joe's brain tell it...you *are* your brain and your brain is *you*.

## Making It Work

How magnificent and incomprehensible the Creator must be who designed such a living wonder as the human mind and body! Is your mind actually you, as Joe's brain would have us believe? Are you *merely* the sum total of your mental activity and capacity—no matter how incredible? You are much more, but let's save that for the next section. For a moment, the spotlight shines on your mind. It will be "upstaged" later.

Picture the following scenario. You are the owner of a successful business. You decide to upgrade your computer system in order to meet the increased demands of record-keeping. Your staff reacts enthusiastically to the prospect. Having a computer capable of handling the billing and mailing lists, monitoring a running inventory of crucial supplies, and doing all word processing will allow employees to devote more time to a matter of greater importance—serving customers.

After considerable thought and planning, you and your board decide to invest in a system of the highest quality. Cost is not the only determining factor, for as Ben Franklin said, "Time is money." Efficient and wise use of time will more than warrant the expense in the long run.

Delivery day finally arrives. The high-speed, main-frame computer finds its place in a special room. Remote terminals, each with a laser printer, set up shop in every office. In no time at all, technicians have the modern-day wonder hooked up, tested, and on-line. You can hardly keep from mentally counting dollar signs. The number of digits makes you dizzy, to say the least.

A couple months pass by quietly and the new system becomes part of the furniture. One day, as you're reviewing statistics from several departments, you realize, to your dismay, that your company's financial picture hasn't improved a bit. "That's impossible!" you exclaim. "How could such a major investment have no effect on productivity?" You decide to do some investigating.

Upon a tour of the offices, you are stunned to learn the reason for lack of progress. Your staff continues to use the new state-of-the-art computer only as an electronic type-writer for letters and memos! "We don't know how to run it, boss," they explain. "There were no manuals and no one has come to train us on it. This is all we could figure out." (Of course, you remain cool, calm and collected as you call the manufacturer to determine why the on-location training team, promised by the salesperson, has not arrived....)

As ridiculous as this little story sounds, it portrays what many people do (or don't do) with their mind. Potential remains untapped because they don't have a manual to teach them. The mind is so vast that even Einstein used less than ten per cent of his mental capacity.

Good news! Your Maker did not leave you to fend entirely for yourself in understanding, or maintaining, the fabulous equipment He gave you. He has provided the Bible, your *"Manufacturer's Handbook,"* direct from the Creator of mankind. In the first chapter of the first book of this divinely-inspired training manual, it says that God, (Father, Son and Holy Spirit), created man in His likeness, as a kind of "shadow" of Himself. After God made Adam's body out of the dust of the earth, He breathed into him the breath of life (His

Spirit). At that moment Adam became a living being whose spirit could worship and walk with his Maker; a being whose personality, mental and physical capacity were unique.

Perhaps you think you're creative. Intelligent. Sensitive. Disciplined. You may be, but imagine this. How would you like to be assigned the task of naming and remembering every animal? Quite a challenge, no doubt. You're not finished yet, though. Now add all the birds...and the fish...and every living thing. Envision such a work assignment! Before Adam's fall into sin, he did exactly that.

## The Mind of Christ

Did you know that you can have a mind better than Adam's? Jesus Christ, as the "second Adam," bought back all that Satan stole from the first man. When you are born again by the Spirit of God, you take on the "mind of Christ." Your divine mind has not fully developed yet, but the seed of the Word begins growing within you like an egg in a mother's womb. Inside that microscopic package, the ovum, exists the blueprint for an entire human being.

The Word of God is the blueprint for Christ-likeness because Jesus is *the Word made flesh.* An apple seed contains the ability to produce apples like itself; the seed of the Word contains the power to reproduce an image of what it came from, which is God. Even mighty oak trees have their start as tiny acorns. Planted in good soil, with enough rain, nutrients and sun, they stand tall. Acorns that fail to receive adequate nourishment die out or at best, grow into brittle, misshapen dwarfs. Likewise with the seed of the mind of Christ. It, too, must be planted in good soil and properly fed before it will bud, blossom and bear fruit.

Through spiritual rebirth and dependence on Jesus, the Living Word, you and I can grow, little by little, to reflect His nature. His heart will be ours; we will grieve and rejoice over the same things He does. His ideas will fill our mind and we will busy ourselves with divine concerns. His plans will be ours. Please understand, this does not imply that you and I will ever be God, or even gods. As long as we are on this earth the old sinful nature will try to regain control.

Beware of "high-minded" counterfeits running rampant through modern society. They fall far short of God's intended best. Nietzsche's motto, "God is dead," has given way to the New Age movement's slogans, "You are God." "Unleash the hidden powers of your mind." "Become one with the spirit of the universe," they urge. Offshoot practices of the New Age include mind control, telepathy, transcendental meditation, ESP, psychic powers, hypnosis, astrology, and subliminal suggestions, to name just a few.

Sadly, countless people are being deceived. These vain philosophies are telling the world what it wants to hear, rather than what it needs—the truth. New-age techniques and humanistic practices engage a lot of mental gymnastics, but they will never produce the mind of Christ. Only the Father, Son and Holy Spirit, through the Word, can supply living nutrients, light and rain to the seed of the renewed mind.

From a distance, psychic activities look appealingly genuine. So also does a plastic, five-and-ten-cent-store variety rose bear some resemblance to the real thing. Silk roses are even more genuine-looking. Until you get up close. What is the missing element? Life. Who has not seen the brilliance of a rosebush in full bloom, watched the play of the wind across velvety petals, or enjoyed the sweet fragrance wafting on the summer breeze? What beauty the world would miss if rosebuds never became roses.

Unfortunately, many of man's present intellectual accomplishments have originated from a mind suffering the consequences of Adam's fall from grace. Without the renewed "mind of Christ" all of man's creative efforts are only self-centered and temporary. Jesus' mind is humble, not proud; serving, not taking; obedient, not rebellious. These character traits should be your top priority goals.

*"Let this mind (attitude) be in you, which was also in Christ Jesus: who... made Himself of no reputation, and took upon Him*

*the form of a servant... and became obedient unto death....*"
(Philippians 2:5,7,8 KJV). "His humility was His capacity— His
fitness— for rising to the throne of God," wrote Andrew Murray. "This mind must be in us if the hidden wisdom of God is
to be revealed to us in its power."[2]

Deep-down motivation for having a transformed mind
is an important consideration. It reveals tell-tale evidence
of the genuine vs. the fake. Knowledge, for its own sake, puffs
up a person with pride. My own life has exemplified this trait
at times.

Pride drove me to study intensely throughout medical
school and beyond to "prove myself." While building a practice, my pride caused colleagues to feel competitive resentment toward me. Regretfully, I have often stepped on people's
feelings in my efforts to be out in front. The Lord always
deals with me about motives. So you might ask yourself,
"Why do I want to renew my mind? To become wealthy and
famous? To have prestige and power over others? To appear
and feel superior to them? To see how creative I can be?"

King Solomon can save you the trouble if you read the
book of Ecclesiastes. He pursued every intellectual, creative,
fleshly feat possible to man because he had the wealth and
time to do so. *"Vanity of vanities,"* he ended up saying about it
all. In other words, don't bother. Those roads in themselves
just lead to deadends. Right motivation for achieving "soul
greatness" is to serve God and humanity—in that order.

# 6. Shape-Up: Thoughts/ Feelings/Will

Once you determine whether you have godly reasons for renewing your mind, you might be wondering, "How do I go about achieving total mental fitness? I know, the Word, but...." Let's review the physical body for a moment. A healthful regimen basically consists of: 1) replacing harmful food and habits with beneficial ones 2) adding strenuous activity to challenge the body physically. A good mental fitness program works in a similar manner. Eliminate what's unhealthy (worry and negative influences from our materialistic, self-gratifying society); add what's healthy, and give yourself enough challenge. (If you have serious mental or emotional problems, by all means see a reputable Christian professional.)

## Intellectual House-Cleaning

Worry is one of the most devastating, common thought patterns of the human race. I would venture to say that most of us suffer from worry periodically, at least. If I don't depend on Jesus continually, worry plagues me. John Haggai's popular book, *How to Win Over Worry,* gives some excellent suggestions for overcoming this sin. That's right, *sin,* and John lists twenty-two physical ailments that result from it. He used to be a chronic worrier, so he knows. Now he follows a simple worry antidote formula that goes like this: "Praise + poise + prayer = peace."[3]

What kind of diet does your mind munch on regularly? Consider T.V shows, movies, videos, books, magazines, music. Are they the junk food variety? Worse yet, highly toxic—like pornography? If so, you probably aren't feeling your best and your thoughts aren't what you'd like them to be. Many men, including Christian married men, are tempted to read magazines like "Playboy." That is, until the Spirit convicts them. A husband's eyes should only see his wife. Lust is an area of weakness for most men; fueling it proves to be lethal. Of course, the pornography industry denies any correlation, but Ted Bundy, mass murderer of young, beautiful women, confessed his lifetime addiction to increasingly graphic, violent pornography.

That's why the apostle Paul admonishes, *"Finally, brethren, whatever is true, whatever is honorable, whatever is right, whatever is pure, whatever is lovely, whatever is of good repute, if there is any excellence and if anything worthy of praise, let your mind dwell on these things"* (Philippians 4:8). Paul understood that you become what you think about all day long.

Picture the following situation. Someone knocks on your front door and when you open it, he walks into your favorite room with a huge, plastic bag in his hand. The next thing you know, he dumps his week's garbage all over your new carpet and furniture. Imagine that! Would you stand there speechless and allow him to continue? Hardly! No doubt, you'd have something to say if he started bringing in another bagful.

Yet, many people allow society to dump anything and everything into their mind continually and they think nothing of it. Isn't the mind more precious than beautiful carpet and furniture? The moral of the story is this: guard what goes into your mind like an armed soldier. Like a Secret Service agent protects the president of the United States. It's just as valuable.

Think about the people you associate with all the time. What kind of diet does their mind munch on regularly? You will be influenced by them, whether you like it or not. The book of Proverbs emphasizes over and over the importance of the company you keep, like *"He who walks with wise men shall be wise, but the companion of fools will suffer harm"* (Proverbs 13:20). In the past, I had a favorite friend who was quite a fun guy, but he was always up to no good. Tragically, he became addicted to drugs and lost his license to practice. If I had allowed myself to continue to socialize with him, where would I be now? "There, but for the grace of God, go I...."

True, Christians are commanded to love unconditionally and bring those in need out of the darkness in which they live. The Lord doesn't place you in a bubble of protection from the world, but you're in the world, not of it. Ministry to others is different from building close relationships with them and doing what they do. Fools, as referred to in the above proverb, are different from those who realize the error of their ways and ask for help.

I have discovered two basic types of people: those led by their desires and those led by discipline. Desires will destroy you. Discipline will build you. If you're trying to become a godly, disciplined person in every area of your life, spend quality time with Christians who exemplify those character traits.

## Intellectual Remodeling

So much for eliminating some elements that are harmful to the temple of your mind. Let's move on to what to add to your mental diet to promote top-notch condition. First and foremost: eat plenty of the Word of God, the Bread of life. You can increase discipline in all areas of your life by committing to frequent, systematic Bible study. Remember, make wisdom (the application of knowledge) your goal and not just knowledge itself—a secret Solomon learned.

Begin by reading the Bible yourself regularly, if you haven't already. Reading in "fits and starts" won't get you mentally fit, any more than exercising every once in awhile will tone your muscles. A version of the Bible broken down into daily, bite-sized pieces may make it easier for you to be consistent.

Try topical studies that interest you, like *"health,"* *"obedience,"* or *"discipline,"* for instance. You can look up any word in a concordance and see which Bible passages contain it. How about an in-depth word study? You may be amazed awhat you can learn by looking up the original Hebrew (Old Testament) or Greek (New Testament) meaning to a word that intrigues you. A concordance, Bible dictionaries, lexical aids and handbooks will become your treasured friends.

Hearing the Word is equally important. Listen carefully to your own pastor's messages, Christian radio and television teaching programs and cassettes. If you take notes, the information will become more a part of you. In my own busy schedule, I have grown to appreciate radio programs and cassettes immensely. When I'm getting ready in the morning and every possible moment during the day, a biblical message is playing. You know what? I never tire of hearing the Word and I always learn something new.

Reading and hearing the Word will lead you to another exciting adventure—Scripture memorization. God told Joshua, *"This book of the law shall not depart from your mouth, but you shall meditate on it day and night, so that you may be careful to do according all that is written in it; for then you will make your way prosperous, and then you will have success"* (Joshua 1:8). If you haven't written the Word deep in your heart (memorization), you will have difficulty speaking it— unless you have your nose in a Bible all day long.

In former days you may have gorged your mind on every form of unhealthy garbage and now you want to renew it. You've learned a hard lesson, haven't you? Your thoughts are reaping the harvest of bad seed sown for years. Well, take heart; there is hope. But remember, a person terribly out of shape physically will not get in optimum condition overnight. It takes time, persistence and discipline. The same holds true mentally. "Never give up, never give up, never give up!" exclaimed Winston Churchill. He helped bring England out of one of the worst periods in her history.

One acquaintance of mine who triumphed over a very destructive past comes to mind as a case in point. This long-haired, bearded young man had literally burned out his brain on hallucinogenic drugs, and used to ride around town on a bicycle with a live monkey on his back. He seemed beyond help. But one day he met Jesus! All he could do was read the Bible and he even memorized a number of verses. Later, I introduced him to an attractive lady at church; they married and he pursued a career in computer consulting. Surely, the Word of God made this man's mind brand new.

Some experts suggest scriptural thought replacement as a helpful technique. Try a simple experiment in order to understand the underlying principle. Think of a black and white spotted cow. Now . . . stop seeing that black and white spotted cow. You probably can't. Think of a brown and white speckled fawn standing in the forest. Where's the cow?

Fill your mind with God's thoughts and there won't be room for the devil's lies, wrote Erwin Lutzer, in essence. It's true. When evil thoughts plague you, counteract them with the Word. Make the verses specific to the problem you're facing, based on Scriptures you have been learning and memorizing during your study time. If you are born again by the Spirit of God and believe the authority of the Word, it will work. Mere positive thinking without dependence on the cross of Christ results in frustration in the long run.

Jesus teaches the same principle as thought replacement, although in the spiritual realm, in His parable of the empty house. The main character of the parable receives a thorough house-cleaning from evil spirits, but fails to refill his temple with the Word and the Holy Spirit. Disaster results.

> *When the unclean spirit goes out of a man, it passes through waterless places seeking rest, and not finding any, it says, "I will return to my house*

*from which I came." And when it comes, it finds it swept and put in order. Then it goes and takes along seven other spirits more evil than itself, and they go in and live there; and the last state of that man becomes worse than the first.*

Luke 11:24-26

As I'm sure you've noticed, consistently *acting* upon what you've read and heard is another matter entirely. The Holy Spirit really becomes your Helper then. We'll save Him for the next section about the spiritual temple. The best always comes last.

In addition to feeding your mind the Word of God—your top priority—here are a few other ideas to strengthen, flex, and tone the intellectual portion of your mental muscle. You might pursue more education in your field or a new one—a high school GED (General Educational Development) equivalency diploma if you never graduated, college degree programs, continuing education classes, correspondence courses, vocational school or even private lessons. Don't forget self-education, like taking a few moments for vocabulary-building exercises, remembering names or simply reading good material. The possibilities are virtually endless.

Be careful, though, to measure everything you learn against the standard of the Bible. Much of the information out there in the world directly contradicts God's principles. When I am in doubt, I ask the opinion of others who have studied the Word for many years, and who have visible evidence of the fruit of the Holy Spirit in their lives.

Another way to stimulate your mind is by increasing your awareness of your environment. Build a deeper appreciation of God's creation—nature and people. I vividly remember how the High Sierra Mountains affected me during the 1982 Western States 100-mile run. Awesome giant redwoods surrounded me and reverberated the majesty of my Creator. I could only express my gratitude to Him as I ran over His land. Such peace was mine during that run. En route, I was even able to mentally complete the third rewrite of my book, *Come Unto Me,* then still in manuscript form.

To daily be more alert and sensitive to the little things around me—beautiful sights and sounds, unspoken messages of pain and need—has become more important to me. I am trying. The hectic pace of everyday life easily causes me to become desensitized. My co-workers can attest to the fact that I still have room for improvement in this area. You too?

Let's move on to another facet of the mind that has tremendous potential to impact your life for good or evil—your emotions.

## Emotions: Making Them Work *For* You

Have you ever known a football team who loses every game? In his book, *Emotions: Can You Trust Them?* respected Christian psychologist Dr. James Dobson tells the story of such a team who lived in a small town in the 1930's. A wealthy oil producer finally made the guys an incredible offer: if they could just beat their hottest rivals in the next game, he would buy every player and coach a new Ford. (Back in the 1930's, that was quite a deal.) The whole school sure got fired up that week. Did it help the team win? No. They lost 38-0!

Dr. Dobson summarized the reason perfectly when he said, "Seven days of hoorah and whoop-de-do simply couldn't compensate for the players' lack of discipline and conditioning and practice and study and coaching and drill and experience and character. Such is the nature of emotion."[4]

As wonderful as some feelings can be, they simply aren't dependable enough to rule your life by. You have no doubt heard the advice, "Never make a decision in the heat of emotion." Yet, millions of people do. Emotions should give way to sound thinking and a disciplined will. If you're a Christian, you have Someone else to be accountable to, as well. Dr. Dobson continues,

The need for self-control is emphasized by the difficulties and stresses that occur in the lives of virtually every human being on earth. As Mark Twain said, "Life is just one darn thing after another." It's true. At least once every two weeks, someone gets a chest cold or the roof springs a leak or the car throws a rod or an ingrown toenail becomes infected or a business crisis develops. Those minor frustrations are inevitable. In time, of course, more significant problems develop. Loved ones die and catastropic diseases appear and life slowly grinds to a conclusion. This is the nature of the human experience, like it or not. That being true, nothing could be more dangerous than to permit our emotions to rule our destinies. To do so is to be cast adrift in the path of life's storms.[5]

What can you do if your emotions get the best of you from time to time? The ones I personally battle most are resentment and impatience. For example, having to repeat myself countless times to patients causes my frustration level to rise. A couple simple steps often work for me. Right before I'm ready to lose my cool I pause and quietly pray, especially thanking the Lord for that patient. Then I can honestly say something to him or her like, "It's not easy, we know. We love and appreciate you, and we're thankful you have come to St. Luke's. We'll try to help you every way we can." Any negative emotions usually settle down.

John Haggai gives a helpful analogy about managing feelings through the antidote of praise, "When rejoicing has become the habit pattern of your life you are not a thermometer personality registering the temperature of your environment. You are rather a thermostat personality setting the temperature."[6] And here's one more piece of good advice from a small plaque in a country restaurant: "It takes thirteen muscles to smile and thirty-three to frown! So why overwork?" (Burn your extra calories on larger muscles, instead.)

The key to dealing with strong emotions, according to experts, is to be honest, first of all. Don't insist, "I'm not angry!" when you're ready to explode. That doesn't mean you blurt out to the nearest available person exactly what's bothering you, "in no uncertain terms." Confess to the Lord how you're feeling before anyone else. He knows already, of course, but it will help you to get it out. Repent immediately. Don't harbor bitter feelings and nurse them. They will get sicker and you will, too (Hebrews 12:15). *"A happy heart is a good medicine and a cheerful mind works healing, but a broken spirit, dries the bones"* (Proverbs 17:22 AMP). That's good wisdom.

Next, search the Scriptures, especially the Psalms, for appropriate verses and passages to alleviate your feelings. Great men and women of faith dealt with painful emotions and you can learn from them. Jesus felt everything you will ever encounter in your lifetime, so you can depend on Him completely. He is the wounded Healer. Pray, even when it's the last thing you want to do. (Your will gets involved here.) You might have to remind yourself that your relationship with God does not depend on your feelings. Sometimes you also benefit by confessing your faults to your spouse or a friend who is grounded in the Word, *"so that you may be healed"* (James 5:16). Don't be afraid to request their prayer support. There is power when two Christians agree according to God's Word.

David Seamands, in his best-selling book, ***Healing For Damaged Emotions,*** says even Christians have past emotional wounds and scars so deep, they need intensive work in this area,

> We preachers have often given people the mistaken idea that the new birth and being "filled with the Spirit" are going to automatically take care of these emotional hang-ups. But this just isn't true. A great crisis experience of Jesus Christ, as important and eternally valuable as this is, is not a shortcut to

emotional health. It is not a quickie cure for personality problems.

It is necessary that we understand this, first of all, so that we can compassionately live with ourselves and allow the Holy Spirit to work with special healing in our own hurts and confusions. We also need to understand this in order to not judge other people too harshly, but to have patience with their confusing and contradictory behavior. In so doing, we will be kept from unfairly criticizing and judging fellow Christians. They're not fakes, phonies, or hypocrites. They are people, like you and me, with hurts and scars and wrong programming that interfere with their present behavior.[7]

Many other experts and organizations would agree. Emotions Anonymous, a growing off-shoot of Alcoholics Anonymous, which utilizes a "twelve-step" program similar to A.A., exists solely to help people overcome emotional problems. There are some sound principles in E.A., as long as one recognizes that the only true "Higher Power" is Jesus Christ. It has been said that the founders of Alcoholics Anonymous were Christians and based "the twelve steps" on the Bible, but time and public demand may have diluted their original intent somewhat.

## Top-Notch Stress-Reliever/Motivator: Exercise

George Sheehan's book, *Running and Being,* speaks of the uplifting mental aspects of running. Although Sheehan and I share different spiritual perspectives, I agree with him about the tremendous relief of tension from exercise. It's joyous! A feeling of freedom is born. The days I don't run, I realize how much I depend on it. I feel more agitated and depressed, and not as outgoing. There's something about the sport that provides a remedy for anxiety and depression.

I have talked to many people about the relationship between running and state of mind. Those who become accustomed to early morning exercises and the stirring of their body metabolism, and then don't work out a day or two, say they have the "blahs." It's true for me. When I miss my two hours of morning exercise, I just don't have the same spark and drive, especially on the days I refrain from running prior to an event. I get much more nervous and irritable. (My staff would agree with a hearty, "That's for sure!") Situations that normally don't bother me, rub me the wrong way. Running has become a kind of "addiction" of mine. However, my habit has proved to be healthy and beneficial.

Although perhaps a childish, primitive thing to do, running is so much fun. I run with our dog and take the opportunity to pray. That time enables me to "get my head together," as I go over my problems and develop a better attitude toward them. Worry—that panicky feeling about everyday situations—tends to creep in during the times that I don't run or engage in other physical activities. When tensions are relieved, I sleep soundly.

As Sheehan points out so clearly, man is a "homo ludens"—a playful one who loves to enjoy himself. It is part of being a whole person. When you take time to play at games and sports in life, you will perform better overall. Dr. Donald Ardell, from the University of Central Florida Wellness Center also emphasizes that wellness should be fun and should lead to a fuller life. Committed athletes get a feeling of "flow," you might say. Everyone who excels in exercise can go through life with a flow and a glow far beyond what they would have otherwise.

In his paper, *"The Second, Second Wind,"* Arnold Mandell describes the psychological-neurophysiological changes that occur with running. He mentions two phenomena. The second wind, very familiar to distance athletes, occurs after about thirty minutes of exercise, and the second, second wind occurs one to two hours out. Dr. Mandell describes these as changes in both mental and physical states.

Serotonin activity, so important for a healthy mind, triggers these changes. Metabolism of serotonin takes effect in the limbic system of the brain, and functions best when you sleep, eat, and exercise properly. Anxiety, lack of sleep, poor nutrition and some drugs inhibit serotonin production.

In the second wind at thirty minutes, Mandell notes that you become more energetic and less inhibited as serotonin metabolizes more actively in the central nervous system. Legs and arms become lighter and your pace, more rhythmic.

Later, after fatigue from the first two hours of exercise, you will have another burst of energy. It is the second, second wind—possibly more energy than after the first one. Instead of just a mental release, you may actually experience a feeling of bliss that goes beyond hunger, thirst or pain. Contentment reigns; colors become brighter; beautiful water sparkles appear and other visual images are possible. According to Mandell, it's almost as if the clouds breathe and the body becomes detached from the earth. Old conflicts seem irrelevant. This second stage of "kindling" is short-lived and again, you will become fatigued. Enjoy it while it lasts.

| Second Wind (after 30 minutes running) | Second, Second Wind (after 1-2 hours running) |
| --- | --- |
| 1st "kindling" | 2nd "kindling" |
| Less depression | Transcendence, bliss |
| Increased energy | Beyond hunger, thirst, pain |
| Legs and arms light and rhythmic | Mental renewal |

Mental and emotional changes that occur during running correlate to electrophysiological and neurophsyiological changes in the brain. Unlike drugs, exercise poses no known adverse mental effects—they are all beneficial. Through exercise you develop your body and mind. First your body, (through the mind) learns the particular sport. As you progress in strength and ability, your mind improves further. Many of the necessary actions and reactions become unconscious and then you can enjoy yourself to the fullest.

Do you have a shy, retiring personality? Through exercise, you may become more outgoing. It gives a feeling of accomplishment, a sense of ability to succeed and overcome. Young people, especially, often have a problem with self-confidence that causes them to escape into drugs and alcohol. Sheehan has found their self-worth develops as they progress in athletic competence. Morale from doing well in a certain exercise activity carries over into other areas of life— creating a positive attitude.

It seems that exercise can help break a debilitating psychological cycle that progresses something like the following one (an adaptation of an illustration Floyd McClung, Jr. featured in his book, *The Father Heart of God:* )[8]

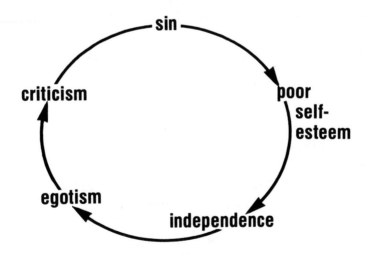

When someone has very poor self-esteem, he tends to become independent to protect himself from people. Egotism and finally criticism set in, which further separates him from others and keeps him from loving and being close to them (and possibly being hurt or rejected). Rebellion ensues.

With increased athletic activity, self-esteem improves and a person becomes just "one of the gang." I have found I lose pride quickly in sports because there are many who can beat me. Certainly, I can't be critical of others because we're all in the same boat.

Exercise not only develops a conditioned athlete's body, but a disciplined mind and challenging, uplifting thought processes. You will be more energetic in everything you do. So, what are you waiting for? If you haven't already, choose your sport and get going. Your mind may argue at first, but later you'll hear, "Keep it up... it's worth it!"

By now we have looked at a number of suggestions to help you deal with troublesome emotions: praise, gratitude, honesty, prayer, group support and vigorous exercise. As we move on to a discussion of the human will, I'd like to close this section with a revitalizing prayer a friend shared with me. (It was written anonymously, but my thanks go to the unknown author.) First, though, here's one last tidbit of "attitude advice" by Richard C. Halverson, chaplain to the U.S. Senate. It's from his meditation entitled, "Perspective," found in his excellent book, *The Word of A Gentleman.* Dr. Halverson writes,

A certain man had been having difficulty with discouragement and depression resulting in some physical disability. He consulted a physician.

The first question the doctor asked him was, "Do you have a view in your home?"

At first it might seem there is little if any connection between a view and depression or dyspepsia. But as a matter of fact, there is!

Perspective makes all the difference in the world to a man. Sometimes a long look at life is the best medicine.

In the midst of nervous tension and discouragement, stop to ask yourself this question sometime, "One year from now, how important will this thing be that is bothering me so much?"[9]

**Just For Today**

Lord, help me...
To remove
  from my mind,
  every thought and opinion which
  you would not sanction,
  from my heart,
  every feeling which you would not approve.
Grant,
  that I may spend the hours of this day
  gladly working with you according to your will.
Help me,
  just for today, and be with me
  In the hours of work, that I may not
  weary or grow slack in serving you.
  In conversations, that they may not
  be for me, occasions of uncharitableness.
  In the day's worries and disappointments,
  that I may be patient with myself and
  those around me.
  In moments of fatigue and illness, that I
  may be mindful of others rather than myself.
  In temptations, that I may be generous
  and loyal.
So that when the day is over,
  I may lay it at your feet with its
  successes, which are all yours;
  Its failures, which are all my own—and
  feel that life is real and peaceful
  and blessed when spent with you—
  as the guest of my soul.
                              —Author Unknown

## Your Will: Strong, Stubborn or Surrendered?

What would you do if you were one of the top triathletes in the world, only to learn you had crippling, incurable spinal arthritis? ***Reader's Digest's*** tremendous article, *"Heart of an Ironman,"* shared the story of George Yates, who heard that unbearable diagnosis. It was during the time he was training hard to win the grueling 1983 Ironman competition in Hawaii

(2.4-mile swim, 112-mile bike ride, 26.2-mile marathon). The pain became so excruciating that he couldn't even stand to be touched. Soon, he was bedridden with swelling and pain.

"Often when Yates awakened in the morning, he hurt so much he had to argue with himself to crawl out of bed. But his competitive experience had taught him that the key to success is an unbreakable mental discipline. He dared not set goals and then fail to try to reach them."

Two years later, after an agonizing training schedule, he finished 134th out of more than 1000 contenders in the 1985 Ironman, walking stiff-legged the last six miles. He went on to compete well in '86, '87 and '88. His greatest goal? To send a "Don't give up!" kind of message to more than thirty-seven million arthritis victims around the country.

"Yates might not be the athlete he once was but he is a far more rounded competitor. 'I used to be focused inwardly,' he says, 'on my accomplishments. Not anymore.' "[10]

George Yates is a tremendous example of the power of the human will. I completed three Ironman competitions when I was in good health— I cannot imagine what he must have endured. Just what is the will? Erwin Lutzer, in his book, **How to Say No to a Stubborn Habit,** aptly describes it, "Your will is your decision-making faculty. Often it is caught between your thoughts and your desires. Your emotions express how you feel; your mind says what you know, but your will tells what you want."[11] George Yates *felt* terrible, *knew* his chances were slim, but he *wanted* to overcome his disability more than anything.

How powerful the human will, for good or evil! That is precisely why God wants it surrendered to Him. Have you noticed that the Lord won't force you to do anything? He gave you free choice because He loves you, and wants you to love Him of your own volition. You alone make the decision to surrender your will to the control of the Holy Spirit. Puppets are not in God's plan; obedient servants are His delight.

## The Battle to Submit

Adam and Eve received divine instructions in the Garden of Eden— only one tree out of all was off-limits to them. Satan "beguiled" or intellectually tricked Eve into disobeying God's will, but Adam knowingly took the apple from her and ate it. Some say it's because his feelings for Eve got the best of him. People are basically the same as Adam and Eve today. An exerpt from *Free To Be Thin* underlines the power of the willful flesh,

> Your flesh, or selfish worldly mind, is something you can control. Uncontrolled, our flesh is wild, unruly; it kicks its heels, rears its head against anything in its way. It is selfish, unthinking, propelled by stupid, meaningless passions. Your flesh has nothing good about it, unless it is under the dominating influence and power of the Holy Spirit.
>
> If your fleshly mind is in control, you'll defile your body at every chance (Romans 8:5, 2 Corinthians 10:3-5).[12]

Erwin Lutzer gives an excellent illustration of a piece of steel (the human will) suspended between two powerful magnets. The only way to completely stay away from the pull of Satan and the kingdom of darkness, is to lean the other way— towards God. The more your will leans in His direction, the safer you are because you're out of the "magnetic field" of the devil.

Truthfully, conflict between your natural human will and God's will is inevitable. One of those things in life you can count on. That's why Jesus taught his disciples to pray, *"Thy will be done . . . ."* Being fairly strong-willed myself, I face a daily struggle to surrender my will. I have learned some painful lessons the hard way. Not too long ago I started a company to provide ophthalmic supplies to foreign eye surgeons. I didn't hire Christians to run it and they weren't doing what they said. Without the Lord's will, I kept trying to get it all to move. End result? The company folded.

Paul was honest enough to say that he just couldn't obey God when he wanted to, and, in fact, disobeyed Him when that was the last thing he intended. He knew from experience the accuracy of Jesus' parable of the vine. Without total dependence on Him, Jesus said we couldn't do anything. Anything of eternal value, He meant. People do manage to stir up a lot of flamboyant activity without Him. My recommendation for maintaining the will in good order can be summed up in five words— surrender it to Jesus Christ. Let Him have it.

When you are dependent on the Lord, then it is He *"who is at work in you, both to will and to work for His good pleasure"* (Philippians 2:13). *"For I am confident of this very thing, that He who began a good work in you will perfect it until the day of Christ Jesus"* (Philippians 1:6). That encourages me. I don't know whether George Yates depended on the power of the Holy Spirit to undergird him or not; the "Heart of an Ironman" article does not say. One thing is certain: if he had, his struggle would have been much easier.

You've read quite a bit now about the mind, or soul, of man, with its intellect, emotions and will. The spirit waits in the wings. Are you ready to learn more about keeping it fit? Good. First, though, let me share one last personal story. You know, as incredible as the human mind is, it is really quite useless— unless it's put to work. We have all probably been impulsive on occasion; I know I have.

My enthusiasm for sports has gotten me carried away a few times in my life. This day in particular I'm about to recount to you has come back to haunt me repeatedly. Twenty years later, people still tease me about my European escapade. As you read, notice the mind's three functions in operation (or out of commission, as the case may be). Afterwards, think about what I could have done differently. Did I do well on any points? How about the other people involved? Here goes....

The setting was Portugal, Lisbon to be exact. Heather and I were house guests of a doctor friend there, and, true to form, I was anxious to keep up my regular running schedule.

Early in the morning I was out the door in my athletic garb. The change of scenery was a welcome companion, so I was enjoying myself immensely as I trotted along. I didn't pay much attention to my route, until it dawned on me...I was lost. Did I know my host's address and phone number? No. Did I speak Portuguese? Not a word. Did I have any money with me? Not one cent!

I kept running and running. The surroundings grew increasingly unfamiliar. Instead of panicking, I decided to just relax and have fun on my latest adventure. After quite awhile, signs for the airport popped into view. *If I can just get there, maybe I can reconstruct my way back,* I thought to myself. (We had flown into that airport the day before.) My logic was right. But retracing our route from the airport to my friend's house on foot took a whole lot longer.

Well...eight hours after my happy departure, I plodded in to my friend's house. Needless to say, my wife, Heather, was rather upset. Our host had long since notified the police with a message something like this, "Officer, my American friend went out running and doesn't know our address. He doesn't speak Portuguese. He probably doesn't have any money with him, either!"

The officer at the other end of the line paused for a moment. Then came his no-nonsense reply: "No doubt your friend will be lost a l-o-n-g, l-o-n-g time."

So, my mind has served me well. Now when I'm out running in foreign terrain I carry a map, wear a wrist compass, and a belt with fluids tucked away— *just in case....*

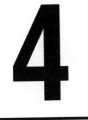

# 4

# LIFE IN THE HOLY OF HOLIES: YOUR SPIRIT

# 7. Just What Is The Spirit?

## In-depth Lessons

"Watch your step!" commanded the guide. "From this point on, we'll be descending...slowly at first, then much more rapidly."

"How much farther down can we go?" my friend, Michael, wondered. "We've come so far already."

"These caves were once the path of an underground river," their stalwart guide informed them. "Listen closely. You should be able to hear the sound of slow-moving water. That is our destination."

Michael stepped slower now, as the path was steeper and a bit damp and slippery. All of the members of his group easily heard the distant water . . . softer than a roar, its crisp, clean echoes filled the air. Around the next bend, the river faintly whispered to them. As his ears strained to follow the river's refreshing music, the guide's voice interrupted. "Before we turn the corner I must warn you. No light penetrates this far underground."

Having gotten everyone's attention, the guide continued, "Just beyond this turn is an immense cavern. Its walls extend upward, outward, and down. At the very bottom, entering in at my left hand and leaving at my right flows the river you now hear."

*No light penetrates this deep?* Michael thought to himself while the guide spoke. The path was well-lit. So much so, in fact, that the brilliance caused the damp face of the rock wall to sparkle like a finely-cut diamond in bright sunlight. Then, as if in answer to Michael's unvoiced question, the guide urged, "As we begin moving to our final stop, I want each of you to put your right hand on the left shoulder of the person in front of you. O.K., get ready. Once everyone has arrived safely around the bend, I'm going to turn out the lights. For those of you who have never been in total darkness, you're in for a surprise. Whatever you may feel like doing, do not move! I'll leave the lights out for only a short while, just long enough for your eyes to become accustomed to the dark. Everyone ready? Let's go."

With that encouraging word, the group filed slowly around the bend and took their places against the wall. A couple feet in front of them was a sharp drop-off. Before anyone had a chance to begin to appreciate the size of the cavern, their guide, after a final nod of his head, put out the lights.

Blackness. A darkness so thick, it defied description, settled over them. Never before had Michael been in the complete absence of light. Listening to the thump—ta—thump of his heart, he sensed a heaviness building in the atmosphere. *How many tons of solid rock are up there over my head?* was the next question plaguing his mind. With that thought, he could almost feel the mountain pressing down on him.

"Now that your eyes have had a chance to adjust, I want you all to hold your left hand about six inches in front of you and look at it," intoned the guide's voice, seemingly from some great distance. Actually, he was only a few feet away, but the darkness strangely affected Michael's perceptions.

He held up his hand and saw...*nothing.* Not the outline of his fingers. Not the outline of his hand. Try as hard as he might, and believe me he tried, he could not see anything. "Being blind must be like this," Michael whispered into the pitch-black blanket covering him. "Thank God for sight." No one responded. *Don't they hear me? Is anyone else there?* His spine tingled with an eerie feeling.

Out of the darkness, the guide asked, "Has everyone had enough? I won't be turning the lights back on yet, but in just a second I'm going to light a candle. Don't look at it. Instead, look around you at the cavern. See how far this little light will travel." Putting words to action, he struck a match and held it to the wick.

The cavern was huge, yet even tiny crevices lay open to the softly flickering candlelight. Whew! All the heaviness of a moment ago vanished as light dispelled the blackness. His small candle lit up the entire place. The darkness was gone!

Michael's childhood experience brings to mind a verse from God's Word. *"The spirit of man is the candle of the Lord, searching all the inward parts of the belly"* (Proverbs 20:27). Just as the candle in the underground cavern brought light to the darkness, your spirit deep within you enlightens your entire temple. When the light shines, you'll see that life-giving river of water begin to flow out to the world.

Unfortunately, when Adam and Eve rebelled against God by eating from one forbidden tree, a chasm opened up between the Creator and the whole human race. Man's spirit sank into the most profound darkness— a spiritual counterpart to the underground cavern. The human spirit could no longer fulfill its original purpose of communion with God. How sad would be the story if that were the final result; it reveals but a portion of the greatest story ever told. Thanks to His grace, it wasn't the final outcome in my life.

The candle of the Lord, man's spirit, was not destroyed when Adam and Eve sinned; its light was merely extinguished. The candle is still there, awaiting rekindling. Worldly, new-age philosophies and practices seek to rekindle the spirit without the Lightgiver Himself, Jesus Christ. (They even consider themselves quite "enlightened.") Impossible! People may develop their human spirit and even become "spiritual." What counterfeit spirit, though, are they contacting? Many spirits exist besides the Holy Spirit of God. The

Bible warns us, "... *for even Satan disguises himself as an angel of light*" (2 Corinthians 11:14). Lucifer (light-bearer) was his name before he was banished from heaven so long ago.

Jesus declares, **"I am the Light of the world:** *he who follows Me shall not walk in darkness, but shall have the light of life*" (John 8:12). He came into the world "*a life-giving Spirit*" (1 Corinthians 15:45), and He alone can ignite the flame of your spirit.

"... *The path of the righteous is like the light of dawn, that shines brighter and brighter until the full day*" (Proverbs 4:18). No longer do you have to walk in darkness, suffering from its myriad oppressions. Jesus lifts the shadows that even the most intelligent, creative mind fails to dispel. Adam, with his tremendous mental capabilities, disobeyed God. The Pharisees missed the mark, and they were the most learned men of their day. A strong, disciplined intellect is essential, yes. So, too, are balanced emotions and a healthy body, but they are unproductive if the will and spirit are not submitted to the Holy Spirit of God.

Do you recall Jesus' encounter with the Pharisee, Nicodemus? Although he was a teacher and ruler of the Jews, neither his knowledge, nor the evidence presented to his ears and eyes, enabled him to see the truth. His reasoning powers hindered his understanding of spiritual matters. Jesus told him, "*You must be born again*" (John 3:3). Rather than accept this statement by faith, Nicodemus tried to question how a man could enter a second time into his mother's womb.

He was trying to understand a spiritual precept with his soul. He had not yet learned the essence of what Paul later wrote to the Corinthian church, "... *a natural man does not accept the things of the Spirit of God; for they are foolishness to him, and he cannot understand them, because they are spiritually appraised*" (1 Corinthians 2:14). Sometimes it's easier to be born again as a child. When I was just seven years old I felt the forgiveness and love of Jesus in my heart and I recognized the power of the Holy Spirit. Later, my intellect tended to interfere when I started "working out my salvation" and trying to earn God's love.

Nicodemus was not the only one who needed to get past his mind to understand spiritual truths. "... *not by might, nor by power, but by my Spirit,*" God had spoken through the prophet Zechariah centuries earlier. He was encouraging His people as to how they could rebuild their demolished temple in Jerusalem (Zechariah 4:6b). The same Holy Spirit empowers you to restore your earthly temple, but now He lives inside you. More effective than mental gymnastics, heady philosophizing or brute strength, He does the work— if you ask Him.

Let's take a closer look at your spirit so you can better develop and maintain it. Like the soul, your spirit has three primary functions: communion, intuition, and conscience. Each plays an integral role, and when working properly and enlightened by the Holy Spirit, your entire temple will be able to fulfill its original design.

## Communion—Getting Close To God

Communion is your spirit's most vital function. Fellowship with your heavenly Father, a walk with the Lord Jesus and the anointing of the Holy Spirit do not occur from far away. They require contact, direct contact. With God, long distance is not "the next best thing to being there." A T & T, Sprint and MCI may offer reduced rates for long distance service, but the only thing you reduce by keeping your distance from God is His blessing on your life.

He created you with a longing deep within your spirit that only He can satisfy. The kind of communion I'm talking about encompasses a "lifestyle of worship"—"practicing His presence" continually. He fills the void in you as nothing else can. My book, *A Heart Aflame: The Dynamics of Worship,* explores this principle in depth. The Lord wants to be more than merely Jehoveh-jireh, the supplier of needs, or even the object of praise and adoration. He desires your total dependence on Him.

When I was in my mid-thirties I was unfulfilled in my Christian walk. Pressures had mounted from the responsibilities of a large practice and an unsupportive family. More than ever before, I began searching for the Lord. I finally quit relying on me as the "kingpin" and learned to depend on Jesus Christ. For three hours a day I prayed and read the Bible and even wrote prayers to Him. Those were wonderful days. From the foundation up He probed my heart, "Are you depending on yourself or Me?" I would like to have been able to answer Him differently than I did.

One other time of intimacy with the Lord stands out in my memory—during the 1982 Western States Endurance Run I mentioned earlier. As I travelled on foot through deep winding canyons, over majestic mountains and across bridges, I truly felt the person of the Holy Spirit.

If you spend time in the presence of the Lord you will want to continue to be with Him. The more you do, the easier you will be able to interpret His voice within you. Like a soft summer breeze, so gentle and quiet is He, you can miss Him unless you're in perfect communion together.

By its very definition, communion implies a sharing, or exchange of ideas. It is not a one-sided affair. Both parties are actively involved in the process. As you fellowship and commune with the Lord, you will begin to enjoy Him. You'll actually delight yourself in Him, as Psalm 37:4 urges you to do.

A relationship with Jesus Christ resembles a relationship with another human being. Time and a variety of circumstances cause it to grow and be enriched to a stronger, deeper bond. Even if you do not yet know anything about Him personally, He knows all about you and accepts you where you are. He has experienced your humanness and wants to give you the means of overcoming your limitations so you might know Him fully.

Joy, excitement and fulfillment will be yours when you have a close relationship with Jesus. Work for it; rest in it and be thankful for that union, the most genuine and productive kind of love. Sorrow, adversities, and trials will come your way, yet times of refreshing communion with Him will carry you through them all.

## Conscience—Let the Sonshine In!

Have you ever done something and then felt uneasy about it? Or, on the other hand, felt an urgency to stand up for truth, in spite of the consequences? A few years ago at a professional meeting on outpatient surgery, I was scheduled to speak on two subjects after the lunch break. At the last moment I felt very impressed to change my talk to an unexpected topic: ophthalmologists were charging too much for their services. (Expense-wise, St. Luke's was in the lower twenty per cent in the country.) In my speech I covered fees for surgery, anesthesia, hospital/operating room, and equipment to patients.

"If we don't hold ourselves accountable for our charges," I challenged my colleagues, "then the government will." Well, you can imagine the response. Many booed. There were strong arguments from the floor and a very heated debate ensued. I was quite an unpopular person that day. But guess what. The government has since reduced ophthalmologists' fees twenty-five per cent and will probably cut them even more. The Holy Spirit was right on, wasn't He?

Conscience, a function of the spirit, is quickened the moment of spiritual rebirth. When the Spirit of God comes to live in you He makes your conscience more sensitive to God's will. You know whenever you fall short of His glory, either with Him or with your fellow man. No longer are outward deeds the only measuring stick of your life. Even thoughts will come under His scrutiny.

Like the candle in the cavern story, the spirit sheds a dim light at first. Disobedience reduces sensitivity, until eventually, the conscience is deadened, *"seared with a hot branding iron"* (I Timothy 4:2). Each successive act of obedience and the subsequent forsaking of sin fans the ever-increasing flame, until it illuminates every corner and crevice of darkness. Watchman Nee, the Chinese Christian martyr, gives wonderful revelation about conscience,

> Conscience is like a window to the believer's spirit. Through it, the rays of heaven shine into the spirit, flooding the whole being with light. Heavenly light shines in through the conscience to expose fault and to condemn failure whenever we wrongfully think or speak or act in a way not becoming saints. If by submitting to its voice and eliminating the sin it condemns we allow it to do its work, then the light from heaven will shine brighter next time; but should we not confess nor extirpate the sin, our conscience will be corrupted by it (Titus 1:15), because we have not walked according to the teaching of God's light.[1]

## Intuition—Guidance from Your "Knower"

Intuition is another function of the spirit. Spiritual "knowing" differs from understanding. For example, a person finds it impossible to *understand* the death and resurrection of Jesus with the mind; he discerns it spiritually. The mind thinks it's foolishness. You do not have to understand something to know it is true; neither do you need to understand *how* a thing works to know that it does, indeed, work.

Many times when God speaks to you, your inner knowing appears contrary, at first, to what you *think* or *feel* is best. He never leads you astray, whether or not you understand completely at the time. His awareness grasps the whole picture. Obey that inner voice; follow the instructions of your spirit and understanding may come later. You will know why God had you go right instead of left.

When I have asked Him, the Lord has been faithful in giving me guidance on many decisions. At one point in my career I was considering going into business with a Christian to set up a division of St. Luke's in another nearby city. It looked like a perfect match. But, the would-be associate was charging too much and I became apprehensive of the partnership. After seeking counsel from prayerful co-workers who suggested against the venture, I decided to forego it. Who knows what heartache we were spared?

Nee writes about intuition,

> To live by the spirit we must move in accordance with the delicate sense of its intuition and depend on its enabling to accomplish the revealed task. Well do we begin if we follow intuition instead of thought, opinion, feeling or tendency; well do we end if we rely on the Spirit's power and not on our talent, strength or ability.[2]

Why, then, was so much emphasis placed on developing the mind to its fullest capabilities? True, your spirit man walks and talks with God, but your mind relays this information to the rest of your outward man. Also, your mind plays an active part in sharing with others what you receive from God. As long as the revelation comes from God and not merely from your imagination or other spirits, He will effect change, in and through you.

## The Spirit in Action

You will always be led to triumph when your spirit follows the Lord's direction (2 Corinthians 2:14). Visible evidence of triumph may take awhile, however. One young couple made the decision to listen to and obey the Spirit of God. Here is an amazing experience they endured, as told by the husband. Look for the three functions of the Holy Spirit at work in their spirit—communion, intuition and conscience.

> It was Sunday night, May 31st, 1987. My wife and I had to be apart for a time and I was laying on my

bed praying. I kept "seeing" the passage in Acts where Saul of Tarsus met Jesus on the road to Damascus. The more I prayed, the stronger grew the impression to turn to that story in my Bible. Finally, when the urging persisted, I opened my Bible to Acts nine and began reading at about the middle of the chapter.

Nothing "clicked." I couldn't figure out why I felt led so strongly to read that passage. Then, deep within me I sensed the Lord saying something like, "Start back at the beginning of chapter nine." I did so, and when I reached the second half of verse nine, it was as if the very words stood several inches off the page. They read, *"And he was **three days** without sight, and **neither ate nor drank."***

I gulped. "What are you saying, Lord?" I kept praying and finally I knew what He meant. He was telling me to fast without food or water, for three days. It was perfectly clear. I couldn't understand why, and I sure rebelled for awhile. The situation I was in at the time was very difficult, and the thought of such rigorous discipline turned my stomach. Even though periodic fasting was part of my spiritual life, I had never gone without water or liquids of some kind. My former pastor had told his congregation once that such abstinence was a "crisis fast." His teaching suddenly came to mind.

After I argued with the Lord for awhile, I surrendered. He was insistent. "O.K., Lord, if You give me the strength, I'll do it. Three days, no food or water." I really started praying more fervently that night, but for what, I didn't know. The next night, it would become all too obvious.

I called my precious wife on the phone about 9:00 p.m., Monday June 1st. She had just come in from grocery shopping, so she changed clothes, and then laid down on the bed to talk to me. After a few minutes she stopped short. "Shhh . . . ," she whispered. "Honey, wait a minute. I thought I heard something. It sounded like glass breaking." She opened the bedroom door to listen, but the house was quiet.

Minutes later, I had to set the phone down briefly to take care of something, so she decided to go put away the groceries. When she got to the kitchen doorway, there stood . . . a man. He was just three feet away. Paralyzing thoughts gripped her mind. *My God, a burglar . . . I'm alone . . . I'm only wearing a nightgown.* Suddenly, the Spirit of God rose up within my wife. Stomping her foot authoritatively, she yelled at the top of her voice, "Get out of here, in the name of Jesus Christ!" He turned around and fled out the back door, with her chasing behind him.

When she came back to the phone she waited for me for what seemed like forever. "Honey," she squeaked, "I did hear something. A man just broke in the house . . . he was in the kitchen . . . I chased him out the back door and dead-bolted it . . . he took my purse and car keys. . . ." Her teeth were chattering so hard she could hardly talk.

I went numb. There was no way I could get home to comfort her.

In His mercy, the Lord reminded me of my prayer session the night before and my commitment to obedience. My mouth was like sandpaper from going without food or water all day, not to mention from fear. When the police arrived, they showed her the back bedroom window the burglar had broken with a ladder. His tennis shoes were still in the dining room in front of the chair where he sat to take them off, just a few feet away from our bedroom. Thank the Lord, my beautiful wife was safe. And believe me, I gratefully finished the other two days of fasting.

# 8. Spiritual Muscle-Building

No doubt you would like to have a spirit sensitive enough to warn you of approaching danger, and strong enough to fight it when it comes. You can have that, and much more. Saying the right words or having good intentions don't count; actions do. Results do not come through osmosis. Wishing without working leads only to disappointment. Many people talk religiously and put on a good show of Christianity—much like the Monday morning quarterback who never really plays the game.

Spiritual growth resembles body and soul-building and is just as difficult, if not more so. Your spirit can be strengthened through a rigorous, diligent routine and total commitment to God's will. The moment you cease progressing, stagnation sets in.

A strong contrast worth noting exists between body and spirit, however. Physical fitness develops after months and years of hard work and discipline, doesn't it? You exercise to strengthen muscles and diet to lose excess fat. Then, after much effort, you enjoy increased vigor and a longer, healthier life. Spiritually, the reverse is true; work alone will avail nothing. You must first receive.

John 3:16 declares that God loved His creation so much that He sent Jesus, His only Son, to provide eternal life for all who would accept. You and I can do nothing to earn His gift. No one can. By a mere act of will in responding to the Spirit's call, you can partake of the promised blessing. Then, with the candle of your spirit alight, you can *"Let your light shine before men in such a way that they may see your good works, and glorify your Father who is in heaven"* (Matthew 5:16).

Over the years, I have practiced four basic steps to strengthen my spirit and enrich my relationship with the Lord. They're simple, but not easy. First, I arise early and read the Bible before doing anything else. Then comes my prayer time—until all negative thoughts and feelings are released from my mind and my spirit is in tune with the Lord. Third, I seek fellowship with others who believe in the sovereignty of Jesus Christ and who are closer to Him than anyone else. Friends provide love, companionship and wise counsel. Fourth, my faith comes alive through Spirit-inspired service to others, both Christians and non-Christians.

## Back to Basics—Word and Prayer

We covered in depth how to study and read the Bible in the section on the soul. If you want your spirit to flourish, you must seek the Scriptures with all your heart. When you begin the day by reading expectantly, you lay a solid foundation for the rest of the day.

Many and varied are the ways God uses to develop your spirit, and every one hinges on the Bible. As you study the Word, your knowledge of Him increases. (Note: be sure your Scriptural diet is balanced with the whole Word of God, and not just one subject you like. Likewise, apples are very good for you, but if they are all you eat, you will soon be malnourished.) And by now, you know that mere knowledge is not enough to live a life pleasing to God. Include the second vital step—prayer.

Praise, confession, declaring the Word, intercession and spiritual warfare, petition, singing, meditation, and listening—are all forms of prayer. These are times when you actively pursue God's heart. Prayer upon arising, before meals and before bed...better yet, prayer in your heart without ceasing!

Prayer involves communicating with God. Meditative prayer, for example, grants the key to unlocking the riches of God's Word and becoming acquainted with Him. With your mind you memorize Scripture; meditating on it allows the Holy Spirit to move the Word from your mind into your spirit where He breathes His life into it. Words burn in your spirit and you know God is telling you something. Revelation comes from the same One who inspired the writers of old. The living Scriptures transform you, little by little, into the image of Jesus.

Meditative prayer involves sharing, the basis for communion. Have you ever seen two people who, though talking to each other, did very little, if any, listening? While one talked, the other was thinking of what to say next. Or, one party could never get a word in edgeways because the other monopolized the conversation. I have to guard against this in my prayer life. Every form of prayer involves listening and waiting upon God. *"Be still and know that I am God...."* (Psalm 46:10 KJV). Without listening to Him, talking will do little good.

One of my favorite Scriptures to meditate on in my spirit is 1 Corinthians 13, the love chapter. Often, as I'm doing my morning run, I'll take each trait of love and bring it up before the Lord. *Love is patient.* "Lord, have I been patient?" Then I wait for Him to respond. (Sometimes I wish I hadn't.) *Love is kind.* "Have I been kind?" *Love is not jealous; love does not brag and is not arrogant... is not provoked, does not take into account a wrong suffered.* "Lord, do I resent anyone who has wronged me? Am I *bearing, believing, hoping and enduring all things?"*

Every time you fail, let your conscience speak to you during your prayer time. Immediately, ask God to tell you at which point you have fallen short of His glory. He will show you whether it was a wrong deed, a wrong thought, or perhaps a right deed with a wrong motive. Repent when that inner uneasiness says repent. *"If we confess our sin, He is faithful and righteous to forgive us our sins...."* (I John 1:9). Accept the cleansing power of the blood of Christ. When you have assurance that you are going the right way, keep forging ahead.

Dr. Paul Yonggi Cho agrees with the importance of a receptive heart in prayer. As pastor of the world's largest church, he attributes its phenomenal growth to the following simple formula: "I pray and I obey." Although he makes no mention of listening, he implies it in his statement about obedience. What works for him, or Moses, Joshua, King David and countless others, will work for you, too.

Value derived from time spent with the Lord far surpasses the time invested. While you wait upon God, cultivating your ability to commune with Him, the Holy Spirit will lead you into other forms of prayer, like intercession. Following in the footsteps of Jesus, the great Intercessor, means you will *"stand in the gap"* on behalf of others. My wife has responded to the call of an intercessor more than I have, I must admit. When God gives you the desire to pray for someone, He will tell you how to pray and what, if anything, to do for them. Rejoice on these occasions. Not only is God developing your spirit; He is allowing you to be an instrument of restoration for someone else. Just like Jesus.

Satan will make every effort to steal your prayer time by trying to convince you you're wasting your energy. "Your prayers do no good. Why bother?" he will tell you. Resist him. In every area and at every corner, withstand his lying tactics. For me it's often a daily struggle to make time to pray, but it's what makes work, non-work. He helps me relax, do the best I can and maintain a thankful attitude.

I believe it was Abraham Lincoln who said, if he had just eight hours to cut down a tree, he would spend six hours sharpening his ax. Prayer "sharpens your spiritual ax," so to speak, and saves much time and wasted effort elsewhere. Paul wrote to the Corinthian church of the necessity for spiritual warfare. Although you live in a body of flesh and bone, you don't fight that way (2 Corinthians 10:3). Remembering this truth when difficulties come is the hard part.

God allows trials so that you may use them the way a body-builder uses weights. They are not meant to destroy you, for with every temptation God promises to make a way of escape. Use adversity to grow strong in the spirit, instead. Step out in faith and forgive. Dare to become a spiritual weight-lifter.

A common expression among body-builders goes, "No pain, no gain." Though not completely true anymore, athletes still realize muscles must be worked with greater intensity, for longer periods of time, in order to grow stronger. Spiritual muscle develops the same way. Expect resistance. *"Beloved, do not be surprised at the fiery ordeal among you, which comes upon you for your testing, as though some strange thing were happening to you"* (1 Peter 4:12). James writes, *"Blessed is a man who perserveres under trial; for once he has been approved, he will receive the crown of life which the Lord has promised to those who love Him"* (James 1:12). The result will be worth any temporary distress.

## Fellowship— Strength in Numbers

*. . . Be filled with the Spirit, **speaking to one another** in psalms and hymns and spiritual songs, singing and making melody in your heart to the Lord; always giving thanks for all things in the name of our Lord Jesus Christ to God, even the Father; and **be subject to one another** in the fear of Christ"* (Ephesians 5:18-21).

Why *"to one another?"* Is it really so important? Yes, vital. Many Christians fail to recognize the significance of getting together with other believers. How much they're missing! Don't you need encouragement? A spiritual battle rages out there against the devil and his forces of darkness, especially if you're a Christian. When your helmet has been knocked askew, when your shield of faith needs repair and the candle of your spirit faintly flickers, you need to be refreshed.

Think back to the cavern deep in the earth—how dark it was. The guide's single burning candle made a big difference, but imagine what two candles could do. How about two hundred or two thousand people bearing candles in the thick, underground blackness? Now that would do some shadow-scattering! There's strength in numbers in the body of Christ, as well. If two or more of us are together, in His name, He dwells among us. Fellowship with others enhances time alone with Him.

Jesus called the church His body for a reason. We need Him, and each other. Eyes can't function very well alone. Hands and feet do better when attached. So do believers. The spirit of each one prospers through the ministry of the whole body of Christ, with Jesus as Head. Why? Because the Holy Spirit distributes His gifts among Christians, as He sees fit (1 Corinthians 12:7-12).

You may have a gift your brother or sister needs, and their gifts will strengthen you. None of us has all gifts, spiritual or natural, continually. We are interdependent. I see this principle a great deal in my work as a surgeon and in our investment company. Surely I could not perform every activity in either area. Some of the office buildings are now managed by Christians whose gifts lie in administration. Of course, a few have been "pretenders," but there are many I can talk to and trust.

The church will help your spirit grow through correction and counsel, even rebuke, if necessary. *"Iron sharpens iron, so one man sharpens another,"* advises Proverbs 27:17. The Holy Spirit often gives confirmation of what He has been showing you, regarding direction, for instance, through other believers, for " . . . *By the mouth of two or three witnesses every fact may be confirmed"* (Matthew 18:16). On one occasion a friend of mine from Oklahoma helped me with wisdom and direction in a difficult "political" situation I was facing. It's easy to get off-track without others around. In other words, don't become a spiritual hermit.

Spiritual restoration comes through the *body* of Christ. I know I speak for other Christians on St. Luke's staff when I say that leading people to the Lord together there highlights our days. If another brother or sister has given in to temptation and desires forgiveness, Christians who are spiritually mature will restore him with gentleness. Through their sensitivity to the Holy Spirit's work in them, they are aware of all their own areas of weakness. Have you heard of "body-building?" There it is, at its finest.

## Fruitful Results!

Scrumptious, juicy, mouth-watering fruit. I love it. You may remember my sharing how I overindulged in eating nature's tasty sweets, to the detriment of my cholesterol level. One thing is certain, though. I've never had too much fruit of the Spirit.

Do you want to know the extent of your spiritual progress? Look at the fruit you produce as the monitor of inner health. By examining spiritual fruit, Scripture says, you can tell much about the tree, or source from which it came, whether good or bad, wild or domestic (Matthew 7:16-18). Instead of apples, pineapple, grapes and strawberries, search for *"love, joy, peace, patience, kindness, goodness, faithfulness, gentleness and self-control,"* all fruit of the Spirit (Galatians 5:22,23).

The spiritual variety is not as tangible as pears, bananas and watermelon, but still evident. Your works and words are two of the most obvious "fruit-monitors." To phrase it another way, check out what you say and how you serve. Both are necessary.

Human nature recoils from serving without thought of personal gain. The soul would rather be served than serve. It prefers to gloat in the center of the latest happening—spiritual or otherwise, and satisfy only its soulish desires. Selfless service is unknown to the soul; it requires a continuous work of the Spirit of God.

Jesus Christ came to serve, not to be served, and to do the work of His Father (John 9:3,4). Spiritual maturity embodies growth into the fullness of the stature of Jesus Christ (Ephesians 4:13), listening and hearing with your spiritual ears and eyes, then doing what He would have you do with a grateful heart. Giving to others keeps the water of your spirit fresh and renewed. Flowing in from the Lord and out to the world, it never gets stagnant.

For years I missed the joy of tithing, giving the Lord ten per cent of my income. Additional offerings were non-existent. When He showed me my disobedience, I began giving and giving in order to avoid being a slave to finances. I gave away a lot I thought I couldn't do without, which fortunately, made me depend less on things and more on Him.

In the end, though, I became an extremist and gave away too much, instead of paying off existing debt. Now I'm coming back in line. But the blessings of giving in obedience have been many. I think of one young church to whom we gave space for a building. The fellowship took off and has expanded phenomenally. To meet some of the members and see the impact in their lives makes it even more worthwhile. The Lord has reminded me from 1 Corinthians 13 that I may as well not waste giving *"my body to be burned"* if I lack love in my heart.

"Your life may be the only Bible some people ever read." Have you heard that expression? I don't know who first said it, but he or she was so right. And it's an awesome responsibility. True service, born of the Spirit of God and carried out through a transformed human spirit, represents God's love in action. Godly works go hand in hand with the fruit of the Spirit and help produce more fruit. People do want to see evidence of Jesus' presence. You may have read this saying before, "If you were on trial for being a Christian, would there be enough evidence to convict you?"

That leads us to the other side of the "Bible-reading" opportunity a Christian provides for the world—the words he speaks. *"Death and life are in the power of the tongue, and those who love it will eat its fruit"* (Proverbs 18:21). The tongue may be the single most important muscle in your body. Conditioned by the Spirit, it brings life; anything else brings death. James addresses this point vehemently, *"And the tongue is a fire, the very world of iniquity; the tongue is set among our members as that which defiles the entire body, and sets on fire the course of our life...."* (James 3:6). As a sort of measuring stick, you could ask yourself whether or not your speech reflects the Spirit of God within you. Scripture says that *"the mouth speaks out of that which fills the heart"* (Matthew 12:34). A godly spirit will bring forth godly speech.

*"But let everyone be quick to hear, slow to speak and slow to anger;"* (James 1:19). Perhaps that's the reason God gave man two ears and one mouth. Do you think He wants twice as much listening as talking? When you do speak, try to make your words positive and centered around the Lord. Offer words that build up the hearer instead of tearing down. Even words of correction and rebuke can be done with kindness and love. (Impatience often gets the best of me, though; He's still working on me in this area).

My wife, Heather, heard a fitting analogy regarding the impact of words on people. A human being unfolds, much like a slowly-constructed building emerges—brick by brick. Words have power similar to demolition balls on a crane. You've seen them. With one mighty blow, they destroy what took painstaking time and effort to build. It's sad but true, that good works can be negated by a careless comment. Ouch! That one pinches me a bit. How about you?

One word sums up all the fruit of the Spirit permeating every word and deed: holiness. Absolute dependence on the Lord causes it to blossom. For years, I put the cart before the horse. I read passages telling me to *"Be holy,"* so I set out to satisfy my conception of holiness. Rather, holiness blossoms from spending time with Jesus and allowing Him to produce the fruit of the Spirit.

Let's complete our study of the spirit with a tremendous meditation on holiness entitled, "Fitness Within" by Dr. Richard Halverson.

As a man's body craves health— his soul craves holiness!

Physical well-being: the sense of fitness— tone—strength—drive—hardness—is of immeasurable advantage whatever a man's work. To be in top shape spiritually is an infinitely greater advantage!

Good physical condition increases a man's efficiency and being "in condition" spiritually guarantees a man's best!

Holiness is not piety—or religiousness—or mysticism—or some other human imitation that so horribly misrepresents it. These human efforts at holiness are a tragic caricature of the real thing!

And they are usually repugnant to a normal man. Because every effort of man to make himself "holy" leads to self-righteousness and pride and hypocrisy.

Which explains why so many good people will have nothing to do with religion. They have been driven from it by those who have a false righteousness: those who are so heavenly minded, they are no earthly good!

True holiness is spiritual tone—fitness— strength—drive—sharpness. It means to be in shape within. It means inner resources and adequate reserve.

In fact, holiness is simply spiritual health!

It is attractive—desirable—magnetic. As men admire the star athlete, so they admire true holiness...when they see it!

Holiness is Christ-likeness! Nobody ever went wrong being like Jesus Christ! There is nothing superficial or weak or stuffy about Him!

If He should appear in the flesh in the average office or private club, men would be drawn to Him like bees to honey. There would be a quality about Him that would make Him the center of attraction.

Of course He'd have His enemies! Great men always have enemies. Holiness will always draw opposition. A man's enemies are often the most accurate index to the man. ("Beware when all men speak well of you.")

But good men—true men would be drawn to Him. Because He would demonstrate that which all men lack—even though they may not realize it. His life would reflect that which every man really wants deep down in his heart. His life would make us aware of the emptiness and corruption of our own.

As the aroma of good food whets the appetite, so the presence of Jesus Christ would awaken our desire for holiness, for spiritual wholeness!

Holiness is the gift of God! It cannot be earned. It is not achieved by effort. It can only be received. Christ purchased it by His sacrifice on the cross. It is not cheap—it is the costliest gift ever offered—but it is free![3]

# 5 PUTTING IT ALL TOGETHER

# 9. ■ Wholeness Is A Balancing Act

## Then and Now

What can the Old Testament tabernacle (consisting of the outer courtyard, the holy place and the holy of holies), teach us about total health of body, mind and spirit? Let's dig deeper.

Like your temple, the ancient tabernacle was an integrated unit, a whole, even though it was comprised of three distinct areas. Whenever the Israelites broke camp they took the entire tabernacle with them, indicating the significance of all its parts. Each area was reserved for certain purposes. The priests performed specific activities in the courtyard; different ones in the holy place and still others in the holy of holies.

The outer court is comparable to your body, the part that makes contact with the rest of the world. When anyone looked at the tabernacle, they first noticed the outer enclosure, a white linen fence around the court which separated the tabernacle from the rest of the camp. When people look at you initially, they see your physical attributes, ideally surrounded by a white "fence" of genuine purity.

Most "social" activity of the Hebrew congregation took place in the courtyard because it was the only part of the tabernacle where the common people (non-priests) were allowed. Whereas the Jews came there to bring their offerings and sacrifices, you *"present your bodies a living and holy sacrifice, acceptable to God..."* (Rom. 12:1).

The holy place and holy of holies remained hidden inside the tent in the courtyard. Housed within your body are your soul and spirit, though neither are visible to the eye. Others can readily discern the evidence, or fruit, of the invisible inner you.

Corresponding to the holy place, which contained three objects—the table of shewbread, candlestick and golden altar of incense (Exodus 40)—is your soul (intellect, emotions and will). You learned that with the intellect you think and understand, with the emotions you feel, and with the will you choose. As important as these faculties are, the Scriptures say not to lean on your own understanding, but to trust in the Lord instead (Proverbs 3:5). In the holy place God gave the keys to make this possible; interestingly, they are the same keys you learned earlier to build up your mind.

The table of shewbread in the holy place symbolizes the Word of God. Eat the bread of life and your thoughts will be transformed by the *"renewing of your mind"* (Rom. 12:2). Sound familiar? When dark emotions begin to run rampant, allow the light of the Holy Spirit (candlestick) to shine into them, bringing them back into proper focus. One remedy will cure your human will: let the fire of God consume it to powder on the altar of incense.

A thin veil separated the holy place from the holy of holies in the tabernacle. Only once a year on the Day of Atonement, the high priest passed through the veil to sprinkle blood in the holy of holies. If sin was in him when he entered God's presence, he died instantly. So great was the people's reverence for the holy of holies, they dared not even go in to get the high priest's body; they pulled him out by a rope attached to his foot! Think of the application to your temple. A veil separates your mind from your spirit, doesn't it? Sin prevents communion with God. Without blood from the High Priest, you are powerless to get past your soulish mind.

At the moment Jesus Christ died on the cross, an awesome event took place. The veil of the temple between the holy place and the holy of holies was torn in two, from top to bottom. From that point on, every member of the priesthood of believers may step beyond the holy place of their mind and enter His presence in the holy of holies—not just once a year, but as often as we desire. That is *good* news.

So then, the Old Testament holy of holies corresponds to the most sacred place of your temple—your spirit. God dwells there! Unlike the other portions of the ancient tabernacle, no light of human making was allowed to enter. Jehovah God was the only illumination in this inner sanctuary. Without His presence, it remained dark. In the same way, unless Jesus Christ rules as Savior and Light of your life, you live in darkness deeper than the underground cavern of the opening story. Remember? The Lord alone can light the candle of your spirit.

In the holy of holies stood the ark of the covenant. Several important objects were kept inside the ark at all times: the rod that budded, the ten commandments on stone tablets, and a bowl of manna. Each has significance in relation to the human spirit.

First, the rod that budded was a reminder of Aaron's dead branch that sprouted new leaves, confirming Moses' brother as God's choice for the priesthood. It was a foreshadowing of Jesus, the eternal High Priest, who died and rose again, and who brings brand new spiritual life to those who are *"dead in trespasses and sins."*

The rod in the ark closely resembles the function of your spirit called "communion." First, Jesus is the only possible way to commune with the Father. Not only that, fellowship with the Lord revives your spirit supernaturally like nothing else can.

What could the ten commandments inside the ark represent, but your conscience? God's laws are no longer engraved on stone for all to see, but impressed on the tables of your heart. The unseen writing within a Christian guides him in all his ways and tugs at him when he strays.

Of course, the bowl of manna, the food that fell from heaven daily to feed the Israelites in the wilderness, is incredibly similar to intuition. When God speaks intuitively to your spirit, He gives an unusual, life-giving word direct from heaven for a special moment or need. You can't store it or it will rot, just like manna. Intuition supplies divine nourishment specifically for that occasion.

Above the ark of the covenant, and between two golden cherubim with wings outstretched, was the mercy seat. As the glory of God's presence descended from the throne of heaven into the holy of holies, it rested above the blood-sprinkled mercy seat. Even today, in your human temple, you are dependent upon the Lord to fill your spirit with His glorious Holy Spirit; you don't conjure it up from inside you.

Time spent in the holy of holies provides a fit dwelling for God's Spirit. His radiance will begin to flow through the holy place of your mind and into the outer court of your body. Other people may not go in the holy of holies to witness the glory of God, but they will notice something different about you if you have been there.

Contact with God! This is the most significant similarity between the holy of holies and the human spirit. In the holy of holies and on Mt. Sinai, both set apart frdom the multitudes, God talked with Moses. He gave him guidance during the exodus years. Your body does not know the voice of God; neither does your soul. Can you see why Proverbs 3:5 counsels against leaning on your own understanding?

## Simplifying the Process

"No one part of your being is enough to be your guide. You do not live by thought alone, or by will power, spiritual perception, physical activity, or by feelings alone. You are a whole person, made in God's image, and no one of these is enough to guide you...."[1]

Balance. That elusive quality holds one of the keys to life—in your temple, the world around vou, even the

universe. Every part depends on the others in order to flourish. Temple wellness implies more than the absence of disease. Jesus, Himself, proclaims wellness as "wholeness" in
Mark 5:34.

Abundant life can be yours. The Creator designed His
children to experience and demonstrate wholeness by a
healthy lifestyle. Anything that takes away from a Jesus-cen-
tered spirit, however, or a mind filled with the Word of God
and a body that benefits from its wisdom, depletes that abun-
dance. The foolishness of the world will reign instead. What
you sow, you reap.

Triangles are an excellent way to illustrate balance vs.
imbalance. I used them in my book, *A Heart Aflame: The
Dynamics of Worship,* to portray an ideal relationship with
God vs. a distorted one. (A triangle of three equal sides
shows a healthy relationship—equal amounts of knowledge
of Him, covenant with Him and worship of Him. Imbalances
can be illustrated with several versions of unequally-sided
triangles.) Let's apply the same concept to your temple.
Think in terms of striving for balance between the physical,
mental and spiritual you. Here is one way to look at it:

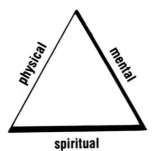

Notice the extra boldness, or depth of color, on the supporting spiritual leg. The mental leg is less bold and the
physical, the lightest, even though all sides of the triangle are
of equal length to provide stability. Without a doubt, the
supremely important spiritual area of your life requires more
depth because it is eternal. *"Seek **first** His kingdom and*

His righteousness; and all these things shall be added to you . . . ." (Matthew 6:33) Give your spiritual life top priority. He who puts God first will be happy at last.

You learned that your soul life, the mental you, is essential, too. Give it priority number two. Realign it attentively, using some of the suggestions I have provided, plus others as the Lord leads you. Finally, your body—the earthen vessel in which your spirit and soul dwell—is temporary, but still important enough to care for with utmost diligence.

## A Question of Authority

Watchman Nee sums up the spirit-soul-body relationship like this,

> Each element has its own particular use. The spirit is employed to know the heavenly realities. Now we are not trying to disparage the use of the soul's faculties. They are useful, but here they must play a secondary role. They should be under control and not be the controller. The mind should submit to the spirit's rule and should follow what intuition fathoms of the will of God. It ought not conceive its own ideas and then demand that the whole man comply. Emotion too should obey the dictates of the spirit. Its love or hate must follow the affection of the spirit and not its own. The will also should bend to what God has revealed intuitively in the spirit. It must not prefer those choices which are other than the will of God. Were these soulical faculties kept in secondary position the believer would make tremendous strides in his spiritual walk. Unfortunately most Christians give them first place, thus eliminating the spirit's position. Is it any wonder that they do not live a spiritual life nor are of any spiritual value?[2]

How about a modern-day illustration as we take one last look at the chain of command that should exist between the spirit, soul and body? Climb aboard a U.S. naval vessel with me for a moment. Salute the captain of the ship—your spirit—who bears the responsibility for the operation and destination of the entire vessel. Outfitted in his impeccable dress whites decorated with colorful stripes, he commands the utmost respect. Under his direction, department heads oversee specific areas of the ship. Usually there are officers of engineering, operations, weapons and navigations. These leaders are somewhat comparable to the intellect, emotions and will of your soul. The remainder of the crew, along with the ship and its contents could be likened to your body.

Once you are born again and have received the light of God into your spirit, you should function like the disciplined crew of a battleship. (A battle rages out there, you know.) Your spirit receives orders from Jesus Christ at headquarters, via the Holy Spirit and relays them to your soul, where the will chooses whether or not to carry them out. If the will agrees to obey, your "ship" will reach the proper destination smoothly and efficiently. In spite of obstacles or danger, every part of you remains on the alert. Otherwise, chaos abounds, as when a crew mutinies on its captain.

The captain, your spirit, is not the only important person on the vessel, however. Where would he be without the sailors who keep everything spotless, fix meals for the whole crew, work in the engine room running the throttle and checking gauges, maintain the navigational equipment or steer the ship? True, headquarters relays to the *captain* firm instructions regarding the ship's ultimate destination, but he would have a hard time getting there all by himself. He needs the other officers and crew, and they need him. The "password" is balance.

## Your Turn

Now it's time for personal inventory. Applying everything you have learned so far, take a look at the following triangles (P = physical; M = mental; S = spiritual):

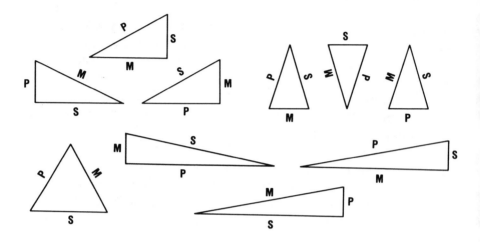

Which one best represents your present temple? Let the Lord reveal the area of your life you have neglected most (shortest side of the triangle). He created you. No one knows you better than He does and what plans He has for you in the future. Doesn't it make sense to ask Him to help you to restore balance to your life?

Maybe He's showing you that you have slighted two of the three areas, to their detriment, and overemphasized the remaining one. Or perhaps you're seasonally out of kilter. For example, every year when I train rigorously for major events like the Double Ironman, it's easy for me to get carried away with the physical aspect. I have to be extra diligent to listen to Bible teaching tapes frequently during that season. Certainly I've never been out of balance with too much Word.

On a separate piece of paper, draw a triangle that *most accurately depicts your temple today.* (It may or may not be as disproportionate as the triangles above.) Finally, ask the Lord to give you a vision of His *ideal balance* for you and *draw a representative triangle.* An equilateral triangle seems best for me, but He may lead you otherwise.

Judge your current state by the fruit you see in that area. For example, are you on fire for God in your heart, but exhausted from dragging an overweight, untoned body around to minister for Him? Or the reverse—have you achieved a healthy, conditioned body, but never find time to pray, read the Word or help others? One more—maybe you're physically and spiritually active, but mentally/emotionally out of control due to a mind unrenewed from past damage. All are harmful imbalances.

Have you ever noticed how much family members affect each other, positively or negatively? If one person feels under the weather, it drains everyone else. Before long, the whole family gets sick because they live in such close proximity. Your body, mind and spirit are much closer and they take on each other's maladies. But guess what. They acquire each other's good traits, too.

If you become more disciplined in the weak area of your life, you will often increase discipline in the others right along with it. Say your weak area has been keeping your weight down and exercising. When you finally allow the Holy Spirit to have control of your appetite and physical activity level (you plan nutritious meals, keep track of calories, make time for exercise), chances are very good that you will want to read your Bible more regularly. Study and prayer times will become more meaningful. Discipline rubs off. Success breeds success.

You can also count on this: anything healthy for one part of you will always benefit your whole being. Your body will be nurtured by the Word. Your mind will prosper from prayer and worship. Your spirit may even rejoice in fresh, crunchy carrots and celery.

## Easy Does It

I would be remiss if I were to forget another delicate balance—the one between *exertion* and *rest*. Too little or too much of either shows you're asking for trouble. Thus far in

*Temple Maintenance* I have emphasized the need for action in every part of your temple. Get moving...make it more vigorous ...build endurance ... develop discipline! Your body, mind and spirit need regular periods of R & R, too. Rest refreshes more when it follows vigorous activity. Work preceded by sufficient rest is infused with freshness.

Dr. James Dobson has this to say about one common deficiency symptom of improper rest,

> When a person is exhausted he is attacked by ideas he thought he conquered long ago. The great former football coach for the Green Bay Packers, Vince Lombardi, once told his team why he pushed them so hard toward physical conditioning. He said, "Fatigue makes cowards of us all." He was absolutely right. As the reserves of human energy are depleted, one's ability to reject distressing thoughts and impressions is greatly reduced.[3]

Remember Elijah after he defeated 450 false prophets who worshipped Baal? That was an enormous spiritual battle and victory. Afterwards, he was utterly exhausted, and one threat from Jezebel— a woman, and through a messenger, no less—sent him into suicidal despair. God's solution for His worn-out warrior was simply food and rest.

Runners do more than race and Christians do more than fight. In fact, if that is all you do, you will soon find your strength running out, your enthusiasm waning and your joy all but gone. Isaiah the prophet gives the following beautiful word of encouragement for living the abundant life, *"In repentance and rest you shall be saved, in quietness and trust is your strength"* (Isaiah 30:15).

God instituted rest when He created the world. Even He rested on the seventh day. You are made the same way. Sleep, relaxation, and quiet time recharge your physical, mental and spiritual batteries. So give yourself a little break after heavy exertion to any part of your temple. You'll be more effective in everyday tasks and have enough energy to undertake the internal activity of life.

Do you ever rest physically, while neglecting it spiritually? Here's a good analogy for spiritual rest—water's symbolism of the Holy Spirit. Think of the last time you took a day off and played in the ocean. Remember how easy it was to splash around in the shallow surf, but more difficult in deeper water? Out where you couldn't touch bottom, you had to rely on your body's natural buoyancy to keep you afloat. Once you just relaxed and allowed yourself to drift and bob along, it was so revitalizing.

As a Christian, you are engulfed in the deep waters of the Holy Spirit. Learn to yield to His buoyancy—His ability to sustain you and keep you afloat on the sea of life. By experiencing this, you can actually surrender to the security of your Provider, Jehovah-jireh, and feel a release from the stress that binds you. The Lord surely understands mankind; He urges hundreds of times in the Bible, *"Fret not." "Fear not."* You, too, will begin to realize that you can trust Him for all things and in all situations.

Abraham had that kind of dependence on his God. Think back to the time when he obediently offered God his long-awaited son, Isaac— his dearest possession. Abraham knew the Lord would give Isaac back somehow, and of course, he was right. That's why he named the spot, *"Jehovah-jireh,"* the Lord our Provider. Trust the God of Abraham. He's the same today. Relax. Rest in Him.

# 10. Yes, You Can!

"There's so much to do, where do I begin?" you might be wondering. Getting started poses the biggest problem for many people facing a total temple maintenance program. Once you've given the Lord first place so He can renew your spirit and mind, simply initiate improvements somewhere—with exercise, diet, relaxation or whatever, and continue to add healthy habits until each area has been fortified. If you've been out of tune for years, don't expect to be a symphony in a month. After all, temple deterioration accumulates over days, weeks, months and years of neglect and abuse.

Remember you're not alone in your quest for total fitness. The Holy Spirit, your power source, transcends any amount of human will power. You are privileged to draw on His power once you have accepted the cost, as well as the benefits, of claiming Jesus as Lord. Having made this step, you are in a much better position to ingrain healthy habits in other areas of your life. *"And my God shall supply all your needs according to His riches in glory in Christ Jesus"* (Philippians 4:19).

## Setting Your Sights

You need a dream. A vision. That clear, long-range picture of where God wants you to be. Anne Ortlund writes, "A dream is a precious, exciting thing that carries you forward from day to day; a goal down the way that keeps you on the straight road to get there, looking neither to the right nor to the left; a purpose just for you alone, exhilarating enough to give you momentum for a long time to come."[4]

That's it! "Exhilarating enough to give you momentum for a long time to come...." I would have to say my life's vision is: to *love* like Jesus. Why don't you spend some time in prayer asking the Lord to give you vision for your life, if you don't already have one? Make a request for your temple, too, so you will be able achieve your life vision. Erwin Lutzer says appropriately, "If you don't believe life is worth living, it won't make much difference to you if you break sinful habits or reinforce them. A purposeful life, therefore, is the basis for discipline and determination to make right choices."[5]

Jesus knew exactly what His purpose was here on earth and you can, too. It will be more specific than just "doing God's will." Noah's vision was to build the ark. Nehemiah's vision was to rebuild the walls of Jerusalem. Paul's vision was to build the church of Jesus. Without vision, you'll be apathetic. *"Where there is no vision, the people are unrestrained"* (Proverbs 29:18). With vision, you'll care a lot and reach higher!

Spirit-inspired goals form the day-by-day road map to your vision. They are building blocks that keep you on track, always moving toward your ultimate purpose, despite failures and setbacks. Consistent progress toward small, achievable goals will reap positive benefits.

John Haggai summarizes goals in his book, *Lead On!* "A good goal-setting program is a S-M-A-R-T one. The goals are Specific. Measurable. Attainable. Realistic, and Tangible."[6] If the Lord inspires your vision and goals in the first place, you can depend on Him to help you complete them.

Consider the following five-part approach to success: "1) Commitment and attitudes; 2) Truth; 3) Goals; 4) Attentiveness; 5) Obedience," recommended by *Free to Be Thin* founder Neva Coyle.[7] She's right, and her five points apply to any new habit you may want to develop. You can have all the good intentions in the world, but unless you get down to acting on them, you'll get nowhere fast. Actions are visible demonstrations of invisible thoughts.

Actions lead to habits, a term I have mentioned a few times now. Do you remember back at the beginning of the book, when a colleague asked me how I developed so much self-discipline in the area of temple maintenance? "Habit," I responded. Let's see how habits fit into the scheme of vision and goals. They should be stepping stones to help you achieve them.

Habits can be either a blessing or a curse, a person's close friends or his arch enemies. The mind isn't picky in this regard. Once you perform an action (good or bad) repeatedly, it becomes a tendency. Soon, automatic pilot is on; your will is no longer involved. You probably don't even give any thought to the action. Eventually, concerted effort is required to stop it. Finally, if you don't check the habit, it will attain a compulsion-addiction label. Compulsive people feel completely powerless to resist their addiction without serious assistance. (Sandy LeSourd has written a popular new book, entitled, **The Compulsive Woman,** and other titles have sprung up out of demand.)

What a fantastic gift habits are, though, when used wisely! Imagine if you had to use considerable mental energy every morning to decide whether or not to brush your teeth, take a shower, get dressed or go to work? You would be exhausted before you hardly began the day. Instead, those activities have become habits. They're easy. Thus, your mind and spirit are free to soar to more exciting, challenging things. Some experts claim it takes just twenty-one days to form a new habit. Monitor the ones you're constantly forming, and make sure they're beneficial to your temple and goals.

Now some advice about fitting all your new, healthy habits into your already crammed-tight schedule. You can't! That's right. You simply can't do it. You have to prioritize your time. After your top priorities are set in place (keeping balance in mind), the other "would like to's" must fall by the wayside if you ever want to achieve your goals. The sun's rays shining on a pile of shredded newspaper will only fade the ink, but focus those same rays through a magnifying glass, and the intensity can start a fire.

Trimming down your activities may be difficult, but necessary. You will be amazed how much extra fat you have in your schedule when you give it a good workout. Expose and uproot the weeds of those old, bad habits that take up too much valuable time. This quote by George Eastman, founder of the Eastman-Kodak Company, may motivate you to practice good time management: "What we do during our working hours determines what we have; what we do in our leisure hours determines what we are."[8]

## Entering Your Promised Land

It's time to march in to claim your "promised land" of radiant temple wellness! Let's say you've already received a God-given a vision for your life and temple. You've written down goals to help to achieve your vision. You're making better use of your time and formulating healthy habits. But there may be one last missing *combination:* a winning attitude.

Joshua and Caleb were part of a team of spies who went to scope out the promised land prior to the Israelites' invasion. Only these two, of the twelve who went, had a winning attitude. They came back with a good report, a willing heart and huge clusters of fruit to show for it. Ten of the spies gave an evil report and influenced the rest of the Israelites to rebel against God. Instead of going faithfully forward to possess the land He had promised them, they resisted. Their doubt grieved Him and caused Him to postpone their entry into the promised land for forty years.

Recognizing their mistake, the Israelites decided to begin the conquest anyway. However, they were motivated by fear, guilt, regret, and anger. More than defeat overtook them. They were massacred. God withdrew His protection and His blessing because they were not motivated by loving obedience.

Why did Joshua and Caleb enter the promised land? They believed God and kept their eyes on His Word to them. They denied themselves, allowed no place for self-pity or panic and acted on the authority given to them as sons of God. Quite simply, Christianity is being "in Christ." You can have this same winning attitude, whether working, playing sports or loving.

A good summary of a winning attitude follows. I call it the *"Christ-Zone,"* a term adapted from a concept called the "C-Zone:"

C-1: You have **confidence** in Jesus. You can do all things through Christ who strengthens you.

C-2: You are **committed** in all you do. Your absolute belief in the Word of God is unshakable.

C-3: You have **control** over every part of your body and mind. You do not let your sinful soul rule your God-directed spirit.

C-4: You are **conditioned** so that your body, the temple of the Holy Spirit, performs assigned work to its greatest ability.

C-5: You have **courage,** the same as Joshua and Caleb, to cross the river and overcome those challenges God directs to you.

These five C's of being in Christ—*confidence, commitment, control, conditioning and courage*—create a new "Type C" personality. (You may have heard of "Types A and B".) Type C people, having discovered their true self in Christ, are characterized by total fulfillment. They have spiritual endurance enough to maintain a winning attitude. "Excellence, with love," is their motto.

One group of people who has learned the invaluable art of a winning attitude, priorities and time-management, as well as vision and goals, are the young Olympic contenders. They must perservere over a long period of time and sacrifice pleasure for excellence in their sport. Several Christian contenders in the 1988 Olympics cited by Focus on the Family magazine seem to have gained a healthy "temple maintenance" perspective about life:

**Jenna Johnson** (swimming, won a silver medal in the 100-meter butterfly; a gold in the 400-meter freestyle relay; and a gold in the 400 meter medley relay in 1984).

"You can't go halfway with anything." Jenna says. "That goes with swimming or your faith in Christ. It's important to remember that we have something much better to look forward to: eternal life with God.

"Before a race, I pray. 'Lord, help me to be the best I can,'" she says. "After it's over, no matter the outcome, I know I've done the best I could."

"I often remind myself that swimming is a temporary thing. It's a gift God gave me and something I can use for Him."

**Suzie Rapp** (swimming, won a silver medal in 1984 for 200-meter breaststroke).

After an injury, she shared, "It hit me really hard and it made me think," Suzie says. "I started asking myself questions like, 'Why am I swimming?' and 'What's the meaning of life?'"

When she realized that her identity shouldn't be found in swimming or anything else but God, Suzie took the biggest plunge an athlete could ever take. She gave her heart to Jesus Christ, and began striving for something that is far greater than the Olympics.

"I'm a child of God and I also swim," Suzie says. "If all of a sudden, I can't swim anymore, I'm still a child of God—and that's what counts."

**Brian Diemer** (steeplechase).

What motivates him to run, bike and swim 150 miles a week in the midst of family and work responsibilities?

"I love to run," Brian says. "God made me fast and he did that for a purpose— the whole reason I'm out there is to give glory to Him." He credits his parents for instilling in him a biblical approach to life, including running.

And his advice for young Christians?

"Set your goals and be consistent, both in your spiritual life and in athletics. If you want to excel, both spiritually and athletically, you've got to keep at it and be consistent over a long period of time. That way, you can be a better witness for Christ and a better athlete as well."[9]

Now at this point you might be thinking, "Well, I could never be an Olympic athlete or a marathoner, anyway." Maybe so. But consider this. Have you ever genuinely, completely expended yourself for a goal? I mean, you really gave it *every ounce* of physical, mental and spiritual courage you had in you? For some of you women reading this book, childbirth may have been one of those times.

Didn't pregnancy consume your utmost? You were more willing to discipline yourself in matters of diet and other habits because another life was at stake. (By the way, a life is still at stake—your own.) Nausea and fatigue may have plagued you for the entire nine months you carried that baby. Labor contractions were perhaps the most intense pain you have ever endured in your lifetime. Was it worth it? When you saw your newborn baby cradled peacefully in your arms, the pain lessened, didn't it? Hurt was replaced by sheer joy.

So many moments of a lifetime are indelibly written in the memory. Sad times are etched there alongside happy times. Crushing blows have plowed their deep furrows in your heart, I'm sure, as they have mine. Oh, but those high points, the "mountain-top experiences" of life...how fantastic they are! They, too, leave a mark on you forever. Of all my temple maintenance memories, such was the Wasatch Front 100-mile Endurance Run of 1982. I haven't been the same since.

Salt Lake City, Utah. Excitement and tension were high. The unspoken question among the contenders was, "Will anyone make it this year?" Not one person was able to finish the last race.

Soon, my young partner, a student from my Sunday School class named Bill Athey, and I were climbing higher and higher. In those days of the Wasatch run, there were no markers to point the way. Only by carefully following clues my companion had traced out on a map the week before, were we able to keep on course. Ours was a sense of adventure. If we'd admit it, we felt somewhat like explorers scouting out virgin territory.

Blisters on my feet began to sting at only thirty miles. Seventy miles left! *Was that snow?* Yes, it was snow alright—light flurries at first and then heavier and more dense, it fell. Darkness enveloped us; even with our flashlights, we could hardly see our footsteps. One other contender continued just ahead, as far as we could tell.

The temperature dropped to near zero degrees. Frigid wind nipped our faces. Still, we trudged on past the sensation of screaming, aching muscles. Prayer, each other and dogged determination spurred us to keep going. *"But they that wait upon the Lord shall renew their strength; they shall mount up with wings as eagles; they shall run, and not be weary; and they shall walk, and not faint."* Isaiah 40:31. More miles lay behind us.

Finally, we made it. Together, Bill and I completed the entire one hundred miles! We discovered that only one other person out of seventeen starters even arrived at the finish line. Gasping for breath, we stood there holding hands and gazing out over the path we had covered. The exhilaration of the moment was inexpressible. It's hard to imagine what heaven must be like, but do you suppose the sweet sense of relief will be similar? We experienced only a tiny foretaste of what it will be like, should we hear those words from the Master of heaven and earth, "Well done, thou good and faithful servant..." Oh, to hear those words!

Tests of physical endurance like the 100-mile Wasatch are great for building the bodily temple, and even the soul. However, they pale in comparison to the spiritual course set before us. Physical exercise profits, but at best, is only "temporary and secondary."[10] Lest all perspective be lost in the shuffle, or an idol be worshipped, our focus is not on health, but on God.

Scripture says the same. *"For physical training is of some value—useful for a little, but godliness (spiritual training) is useful and of value in everything and in every way, for it holds promise for the present life and also for the life which is to come"* (1 Timothy 4:8, AMP). No matter what you do to maintain your outer man, it still gradually perishes. Only your inner man, as the apostle Paul said, will last through eternity.

## Parting Thoughts

Through dependence upon Jesus Christ, countless people endure physical, mental and spiritual burdens that would be otherwise unbearable. They persist and emerge victorious against all possible odds. Who can comprehend the sweet sense of relief at the finish line like they do? They are the *real* overcomers.

The blind and deaf. Paraplegics and quadriplegics. Cerebral palsy victims. Burn patients. The emotionally, physically and sexually-abused. Handicapped children who struggle their little hearts out in the Special Olympic Games...the list continues. No doubt you have known some overcomers in your lifetime. I have, too, and I'm a better person for it. Maybe you *are* an overcomer. Well, God bless you.

I had the privilege to see one extraordinary endurance hero at the 1988 Ironman Triathlon in Hawaii. He, too, completed the course of a 2.4-mile swim, 112-mile bike ride and a 26.2-mile run, and was honored with a special finisher's medal for his effort. After you've read this man's story found in a letter from Help Hospitalized Veterans in San Diego, you'll better understand what I mean when I say "endurance hero."

And if *he* can overcome, so can you. *Yes, you **can!***

Dear Fellow American,

. . . Out on "my mission" crossing the Arizona desert on my way to Washington, D.C. The heat was awesome, bouncing off the desert highway, blasting my face and body. But I made it. It took me 3 years, 8 months, 6 days and some 4,900,016 "steps" to cover the 2,784 miles from California to Washington D.C. . . . but I made it. And that's what's important: I wanted to show that through faith in God and dedication, there's nothing a person can't achieve.

But now I need your help—not for me, but for over 83,000 American veterans still in the hospital. For them, the challenge is not walking across the country on their hands. . . . Rather, for many hospitalized veterans the biggest challenge is simply sitting up in bed, feeding themselves, or just finding the will to live. I know, because I was one of them myself after my legs got blown off in Vietnam . . . .

I still remember what happened like it was yesterday. In fact, it was June 14, 1969, when our 25th Infantry Division unit walked into a mine field. The next thing I knew, mines were going off right and left, killing and wounding men all around me. As a combat medic, I ran to the aid of my fallen buddies. That's when it happened: I stepped on an 82mm mortar round powerful enough to blow up a tank. I went flying in one direction, and my legs went flying in another. When the doctors first saw me, they pronounced me "Dead on Arrival." With the help of God, however, the doctors managed to save me.

I had gone into combat a 6-foot, 200-pound pitcher with excellent prospects of being signed to a professional baseball contract. When I left Vietnam, I was 2 feet 10 1/2 inches tall and weighed 87 pounds. Still, I consider myself blessed. My best friend, whom I was trying to help that day in Vietnam, is now at Wall 22 West, line 47 on the Vietnam Memorial in Washington, D.C.

When I got to the hospital and woke up, I was wracked with pain I can't even describe and too weak even to sit up in bed. But I still had two things going for me: First, I had the greatest anesthesiologist of them all . . . the Lord Jesus Christ, working with me. Lovingly, he spared me the bitter thoughts that many veterans still have.

And second, I took advantage of physical therapy. For my therapy, I worked on my two remaining limbs, my arms, lifting weights slowly at first, then with more confidence. And it paid off: I was able to be totally independent after a period of two months and soon began entering weight-lifting competitions. On four different occasions, by the grace of God, I broke the world record in the bench press.

But still, I felt the Lord had spared my life for something greater, something that would help others. That's when I set out in 1982 on the Spirit of America "Walk for Hunger," walking across America on my hands. It was slow going, covering only 3 to 5 miles per day. It was a tremendously physical and spiritual experience.

I hope my cross-country journey helps inspire you . . . .

With Faith and Determination,


Bob Wieland[11]

*"Therefore, since we are surrounded by so great a cloud of witnesses (who have borne testimony of the Truth), let us strip off and throw aside every encumbrance—unnecessary weight—and the sin which so readily (deftly and cleverly) clings to and entangles us, and let us run with patient endurance and steady and active persistence the appointed course of the race that is set before us,*

*Looking away (from all that will distract) to Jesus, Who is the Leader and the Source of our faith (giving the first incentive for our belief) and is also its Finisher, (bringing it to maturity and perfection). He, for the joy (of obtaining the prize) that was set before Him, endured the cross. . . . "*

Hebrews 12:1,2a (AMP)

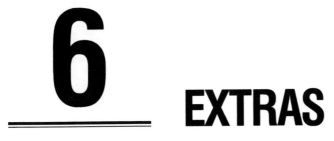

# 6 EXTRAS

# 11. Notes

**Part Two  The Outer Court: Your Body**

1 Randy Padawer, Reprinted with permission from the March 1989 *Reader's Digest.* Copyright (c) 1989 by The Reader's Digest Assn., Inc.
2 Gabe Mirkin, M.D., *Getting Thin* (Boston: Little, Brown and Co., Inc., (c) 1983 by Gabe Mirkin), p. 211. Reprinted by permission of Little, Brown, and Co.
3 Dr. Mary Ruth Swope, *Are You Sick & Tired of Feeling Sick & Tired?* (Springdale, PA: Whitaker House, (c) 1984 by Dr. Mary Ruth Swope), pp. 5,6. Reprinted by permission.

**Part Three  The Holy Place: Your Mind**

1 *Webster's New Twentieth Century Dictionary,* Unabridged Second Edition. (New York: Simon & Schuster, 1983), p. 1144. Reprinted by permission.
2 Andrew Murray, *Be Perfect* (Springdale, PA: Whitaker House, 1982), p. 61.
3 John Haggai, *How To Win Over Worry* (Eugene, OR: Harvest House Publishers, 1987), p. 35. Reprinted by permission.
4 Dr. James Dobson, *Emotions: Can You Trust Them?* (Ventura, CA: Regal Books, 1980), p. 6. Reprinted by permission.

5 Dr. James C. Dobson, **Straight Talk To Men And Their Wives** (Waco, TX: Word Incorporated, 1984), pp. 186-187.

6 John Haggai, op. cit. p. 42.

7 David Seamands, **Healing For Damaged Emotions** (Wheaton, IL: Victor Books, A Division of SP Publications, 1981), pp. 12-13. Reprinted by permission.

8 Floyd McClung, Jr., **The Father Heart Of God** (Eugene, OR: Harvest House Publishers, 1985), p. 45. Reprinted by permission.

9 Richard C. Halverson, **The Word Of A Gentleman** (Grand Rapids: Zondervan Publishing House, 1983), p. 11. Reprinted by permission.

10 Excerpted with permission from "Heart of an Ironman" by John G. Hubbell, (**Reader's Digest,** March 1989). Copyright (c) 1989 by The Reader's Digest Assn., Inc.

11 Erwin W. Lutzer, **How To Say No To A Stubborn Habit** (Wheaton, IL: Victor Books, A Division of S.P. Publications, 1979), p. 98. Reprinted by permission.

12 Marie Chapian & Neva Coyle, **FREE TO BE THIN**, (Minneapolis, MN: Bethany House Publishers, 1979), p. 31. Reprinted by permission.

**Part Four  The Holy of Holies— Your Spirit**

1 Watchman Nee, **The Spiritual Man,** 3 vols. (New York: Christian Fellowship Publishers, 1968; Combined Edition, 1977), vol. 2, pp. 113-114. Reprinted by permission.

2 Ibid, p. 31.

3 Richard C. Halverson, op. cit. pp. 19-20.

**Part Five  Putting It All Together**

1 Erwin W. Lutzer, op. cit. p. 87.

2 Watchman Nee, op. cit. p. 93.

3 Dr. James Dobson, **Emotions: Can You Trust Them?** op. cit. p. 119.

4 Anne Ortlund, **Disciplines of the Beautiful Woman** (Waco, TX: Word, Incorporated, 1984), p. 50. Reprinted by permission.

5 Erwin W. Lutzer, op. cit. p. 101.

6 John Haggai, **Lead On!** (Waco, TX: Word, Incorporated, 1986), p. 43. Reprinted by permission.

7 Neva Coyle, **FREE TO BE THIN STUDY GUIDE #1** (Minneapolis: Bethany House Publishers, 1981), p. 31. Reprinted by permission.

8 Reprinted with permission from the March 1989 **Reader's Digest.** Copyright (c) 1989 by The Reader's Digest Assn., Inc. Also by permission of Eastman-Kodak Company.

9 "Countdown to Seoul," *Focus on the Family Magazine,* September 1988, pp.2-5. Excerpted by permission.

10 "Pumping Spiritual Iron" (cassette), Pastor Bill Anderson, Calvary Baptist Church, Clearwater, FL.

11 Fund-raising letter from *Help Hospitalized Veterans,* San Diego, CA. Excerpted by permission of General Manager, Mike Lynch.

# 12. Bibliography

For further reading on the body (diet):

Brody, Jane. *Jane Brody's Good Food Book— Living the High-Carbohydrate Way.* New York: W.W. Norton & Company, 1985.

Brown, W. Virgin, M.D. and Wahida Karmally. *Making the Break With Cholesterol, Rx Being Well.* January/February, 1987.

Chapian, Marie and Neva Coyle. **FREE TO BE THIN.** Minneapolis: Bethany House Publishers, 1979.

Cooper, Kenneth. *Controlling Cholesterol.* New York: Bantam Books, 1988.

Mirkin, Gabe, M.D. *Getting Thin.* Boston: Little, Brown & Company, 1983.

Pauling, Linus. *How to Live Longer and Feel Better.* New York: W.H. Freeman and Company, 1986.

Pritikin, Nathan. *Diet for Runners.* New York: Simon & Schuster, 1985.

_____ *The Pritikin Promise: 28 Days to a Longer, Healthier Life.* New York: Simon & Schuster, 1983.

Swope, Dr. Mary Ruth. *Are You Sick and Tired of Feeling Sick and Tired?* Springdale, PA: Whitaker House, 1984.

U.S. Department of Health and Human Services. *Cholesterol Counts: Steps for Lowering Your Patient's Blood Cholesterol.* Public Health Service, National Institute of Health. Publication #85-2699, 1985.

Williams, Sue Rodwell. *Nutrition and Diet Therapy.* St. Louis: Times Mirror/Mosby College Publishing, 1985.

Wunderlich, Elinor, R.N. *Easy Whole-Food Recipes.* St. Petersburg, FL: Johnny Reads, Inc., 1980.

Wunderlich, Ray C. Jr., M.D. *Diet: The Process of Change.* St. Petersburg, FL: Ray C. Wunderlich, Jr., M.D.

___ *Fatigue: What Causes It, What It Does To You, What You Can Do About It.* St. Petersburg, FL: Johnny Reads, Inc., 1976.

___ *Patient Orientation.* St. Petersburg, FL: Ray C. Wunderlich, Jr., M.D.

___ *Stress and Its Relation to Diet and Nutrition.* St. Petersburg, FL: Ray C. Wunderlich, Jr., M.D.

___ *Sugar and Your Health,* St. Petersburg, FL: Good Health Publications, Johnny Reads, Inc., 1982.

For further reading on the body (exercise):

Cooper, Kenneth H., M.D., M.P.H. *The Aerobics Program For Total Well-Being.* New York: Bantam Books, Inc., 1983.

___ *Running Without Fear.* New York: M. Evans and Company, Inc., 1985.

Cooper, Kenneth H., M.D., M.P.H. and Mildred Cooper. *The New Aerobics For Women.* New York: Bantam Books, Inc., 1988.

Counsilman, James E. *Competitive Swimming Manual for Coaches and Swimmers.* Bloomington, IN: Counsilman Co., Inc., 1977.

___ *The Science of Swimming.* Englewood Cliffs, NJ: Prentice-Hall, Inc., 1968.

Darden, Ellington, PhD. *Nautilus Bodybuilding Book.* Chicago: Contemporary Books, Inc., 1982.

___ *The Nautilus Advanced Bodybuilding Book.* New York: Simon & Schuster, 1984.

The Editors of Bicycling Magazine. *Best Bicycle Tours.* Emmaus, PA: Rodale Press, Inc., 1980.

The Editors of Runner's World. *The Complete Runner.* Mountain View, CA: Runner's World Books, 1974.

___ *The Complete Runner, Volume Two.* Mountain View, CA: Runner's World Books, 1982.

___ *From the Experts: Training Smart.* Emmaus, PA: Rodale Press, Inc., 1986.

___ *Weight Training For Runners.* Emmaus, PA: Rodale Press, Inc., 1986.

Gipe, George. *The Great American Sports Book.* Garden City, NY: Doubleday & Company, Inc., 1978.

Johnson, Bob and Patricia Bragg, Ph.D. *The Complete Triathlon Distance Training Manual.* Santa Barbara, CA: Health Science, 1982.

Knight, Peter O., M.D. "Exercise and Health," Hillsborough County Medical Association Bulletin. April, 1982.

Lawrence, Ronald M., M.D., Ph.D. and Sandra Rosenzweig. *Going the Distance: The Right Way to Exercise for People Over 40.* Los Angeles: Jeremy P. Tarcher, Inc., 1987.

Rodgers, Bill. *Marathoning.* New York: Simon & Schuster, 1980.

Sheehan, Dr. George. *Running & Being—The Total Experience.* New York: Warner Books, Inc., 1978.

The Surgeon General's Report on Health Promotion and Disease Prevention. "Healthy People." Washington, D.C., 1979.

Sweetgall, Robert. *Fitness Walking.* New York: Putnam Publishing Group, 1985.

Sweetgall, Robert and John Digman. *The Walker's Journal.* Newark, DE: Creative Walking, Inc., 1986.

For further reading on soul and spirit:

*The Bible,* All Versions.

Dobson, Dr. James. *Emotions: Can You Trust Them?* Ventura, CA: Regal Books, 1980.

___ *Straight Talk to Men and Their Wives.* Waco, TX: Word, Inc., 1984.

Haggai, John. *How To Win Over Worry.* Eugene, OR: Harvest House Publishers, 1987.

_____ *Lead On!* Waco, TX: Word, Inc., 1986.

Halverson, Richard C. *The Word of A Gentleman.* Grand Rapids: Zondervan Publishing House, 1983.

Lutzer, Erwin W. *How To Say No To A Stubborn Habit.* Wheaton, IL: Victor Books, 1979.

McClung, Floyd Jr. *The Father Heart of God.* Eugene, OR: Harvest House Publishers, 1985.

Murray, Andrew. *Be Perfect.* Springdale, PA: Whitaker House, 1982.

Nee, Watchman. *The Spiritual Man,* 3 vols. New York: Christian Fellowship Publishers, 1968; Combined Edition, 1977.

Ortlund, Anne. *Disciplines of the Beautiful Woman.* Waco, TX: Word, Inc., 1984.

Seamands, David. *Healing For Damaged Emotions.* Wheaton, IL: Victor Books, 1981.

# 13. About the Author

As an ultra-distance athlete, James P. Gills, M.D., has participated in a total of forty-six marathons, including nineteen of the famed Boston Marathon. He has competed in fourteen 100-mile mountain runs (he's one of only a few dozen people to complete all four major 100-mile mountain runs) and in three 200-mile runs through the rolling hills of Virginia. In addition, Dr. Gills has completed five Ironman Triathlons in Hawaii, as well as being the only person to complete six Double Ironman Triathlons in less than thirty hours. The Double Ironman consists of a 4.8-mile swim, a 224-mile bike ride and a 52.4-mile run. Since 1991, he has "retired" from running, and now focuses his energy on biking, swimming, windsurfing and golf. His passion for fitness has led him, along with his son, to write *Temple Maintenance,* in which he describes the importance of physical, mental and spiritual conditioning.

Dr. Jim Gills is the founder and medical director of St. Luke's Cataract and Laser Institute in Tarpon Springs, Florida. Internationally respected as a cataract surgeon, he has performed more cataract extractions and lens implantations than anyone else in the world. He has pioneered many advancements in the field of ophthalmology that make cataract surgery safer and easier for patients.

Dr. Gills has published over ninety medical papers and contributed to six books, while being an active author on spiritual topics, as well. He has been an avid student of the Bible for many years and has written a number of books about man's relationship with God. (See listing of titles and descriptions at the front.)

Dr. Gills is a former member of the Board of Trustees of Trinity College and of the national Board of Directors of the Fellowship of Christian Athletes. He is also recognized in the Marquis **Who's Who** and many other similar publications.

He is on the board of the Duke University Medical Center and the Wilmer Institute at Johns Hopkins. He was voted one of the Best Doctors in America in 1994 and was asked to present the highly esteemed INNOVATOR'S LECTURE at the 1996 symposium of the American Society of Cataract and Refractive Surgery (ASCRS). In 1990, he was named Entrepreneur of the Year for the State of Florida.

# 14. How You Can Help

**L**OVE PRESS has provided this book at no initial charge, via LoveLines: The Honor Innovation™. Donations will help produce additional LoveLines materials and enable LOVE PRESS to distribute them at no charge. *Most important, please remember us in your prayers!*

Did you enjoy this LoveLines™ book?
Dr. & Mrs. James P. Gills would love to hear
from you! Please respond if this book has made an
impact on you or someone you know.

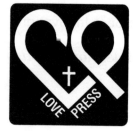

**LOVE PRESS**
St. Luke's Building
43309 U.S 19 North ▪ P.O. Box 5000
Tarpon Springs, Florida 34688-5000
Phone: (727) 938-2020, Ext. 2200
Call Toll-Free: 1-800-282-9905, Ext. 2200